Easy-To-Follow Workouts for Seniors—Master Resistance Band Exercises

Elevate Balance, Strengthen Flexibility, and Enhance Well-Being from the Comfort of Home

Sylvia Silverstep

Copyrights

First published by Global One Books LLC October 2023

Copyright © 2023 by Global One Books LLC

All rights reserved. No part of this publication may be reproduced, stored, or transmitted in any form or by any means, electronic, mechanical, photocopying, recording, scanning, or otherwise, without written permission from the publisher. It is illegal to copy this book, post it to a website, or distribute it by any other means without permission.

Global One Books LLC asserts the moral right to be identified as the author of this work.

Designations used by companies to distinguish their products are often claimed as trademarks. All brand names and product names used in this book and on its cover are trade names, service marks, trademarks, and registered trademarks of their respective owners. The publishers and the book are not associated with any product or vendor mentioned in this book. None of the companies referenced within the text have endorsed the book.

First edition

CHAPTER 4: STRENGTHENING MUSCLES FOR BETTER POSTURE AND MOBILITY 47

Introduction

"Aging is an extraordinary process where you become the person you always should have been." — David Bowie.

Do you remember the ease of climbing stairs two at a time or lifting all your grocery bags in one go? And now, you are contemplating each step as if it's a mini Everest. I've been in your shoes, or should I say orthopedic sandals? Aging hit me like a freight train.

One minute, I'm out jogging; the next, I calculate the risks of bending down to tie my shoelaces.

Your problem isn't just yours alone; it's a universal rite of passage. Mobility is decreasing, balance feels off, and the idea of an exercise routine seems daunting. The worst part? The loss of confidence sneaks in, eroding the freedom to do even simple activities that once felt effortless.

Here's the silver lining: this book is the lifeline you've been waiting for. It's packed with actionable, easy-to-follow exercises using resistance bands—those nifty, stretchy loops that can transform your living room into a fitness center. You'll find routines to improve your balance, strength, flexibility, and well-being.

My mistakes? They've been the steppingstones to the expertise I now share. And not to brag, but my newfound strength and mobility have given me back a piece of my youth.

But it's not just about me. I've seen firsthand how these techniques have improved the lives of countless others. Friends and acquaintances, once skeptical, now swear by these exercises. Their transformation is a testament to the effectiveness of the resistance band workouts you're about to dive into.

This isn't another generic fitness book that gathers dust on your shelf. This is a practical guide with step-by-step instructions designed specifically for you. After soaking up the wisdom packed into these pages, you'll have the tools to reclaim your physicality and the freedom that comes with it.

The clock is ticking, and there's no better time than now to take action. Understanding your body's needs at this phase of life is crucial. No more fumbling in the dark; this book is your illuminated path. You'll soon find that age is merely a number, but well-being is timeless.

Are you cheered up to reclaim some of that old spark and feel more secure in your body? Keep reading because you're in for a transformative experience.

Chapter 1: Aging Gracefully

THE CHALLENGES OF AGING

"Do not regret growing older. It's a privilege denied to many." — Unknown

So, here we are, at a stage in life where the words "aging gracefully" are more than just a throwaway line at family gatherings. We've all felt it—the creak in the knees as you get up from a chair, the stiffness in the back that wasn't there a decade ago, and even the mirror seems a bit less forgiving these days.

In the spirit of full disclosure, I've been there. I've felt that twinge of uncertainty before stepping onto an escalator, worried about whether my balance could hold up. I've had those mornings where my joints decided to play their cacophony, each crack and pop a reminder of the years gone by. Aging is not for the faint-hearted, and while we can't stop the clock, we can undoubtedly negotiate better terms with time.

One of the most challenging aspects of aging is the loss of physical abilities that used to be second nature. For instance, remember when you could bend down to pick up a dropped pen without a second thought? Now, that simple action requires a mental pep talk. And let's not even talk about the herculean effort it takes to put on socks in the morning. These small but impactful changes are the nitty-gritty details that don't make it into the "Golden Years" brochure.

However, the challenges aren't just physical and spill over into the emotional realm. A mental toll comes with feeling less capable, a shadow that can cloud even the sunniest disposition. You start to decline invitations to social events out of fear that there'll be stairs or, worse, dancing. The mental calisthenics required to navigate what used to be simple daily tasks can be exhausting.

You might wonder, "Why is this book digging into all these uncomfortable truths?" Well, because the first step to solving a problem is acknowledging it. We're not here to wallow in the setbacks but to rise above them. Enter resistance bands—your soon-to-be partners in crime for tackling these challenges head-on.

For the skeptics out there, I get it. It's easy to dismiss something as too good to be true. But remember, I've walked this path. I've felt the limitations and frustrations. I tried countless exercise regimes before stumbling upon resistance bands; the difference was night and day. The simplicity, the low risk of injury, and the tangible results made me believe. And that's why I wrote this book—to share this highly effective approach to overcoming the physical challenges of aging.

Here's the deal: I can't offer you a time machine, but I can provide the next best thing—a way to make the most of the time you have. The exercises in this book are more than just a series of movements; they're a lifeline to a better quality of life. They focus on the core issues we face as we age—balance, strength, flexibility, and, yes, even confidence.

THE POWER OF SENIOR FITNESS

"Age is merely the number of years the world has been enjoying you. Cheers to you and your contribution to making the world a more beautiful place." — Unknown

---

Getting older is often associated with a decline in physical abilities. But here's the truth bomb: age is just a number for fitness. The real magic lies in the mindset and the willingness to stay active, irrespective of the candles on your birthday cake. So, if you're thinking it's too late to get fit, scrap that thought right now. The benefits of fitness, especially in the senior years, are nothing short of transformative.

Firstly, let's talk about the elephant in the room: the myth that fitness and age are inversely proportional. People often believe that their fitness levels will plummet as they age. But hold on a minute! Several studies have shown that regular physical activity can significantly improve muscle strength and endurance, even in older adults. You might not sprint like a 20-year-old, but you can build enough stamina to enjoy long walks without panting for breath.

Secondly, let's discuss mobility. One of the most frustrating aspects of aging can be the loss of mobility. It's not just about being able to run or jump but about doing simple things like tying your shoes or reaching for a jar on the top shelf. Fitness routines designed for seniors often focus on improving the range of motion. The beauty of this is that it translates into everyday activities, making you more independent and agile.

Now, let's talk about mental health. There's an undeniable link between physical and psychological well-being. Regular exercise can drastically improve your mental health by reducing symptoms of depression and anxiety. The endorphins released during physical activity act as natural mood lifters. So, fitness doesn't just make you stronger physically; it also acts as a natural antidepressant.

A mention of bone health is a must here. One of the hidden benefits of senior fitness is its positive impact on bone density. Our bones become more brittle as we age, making us more susceptible to fractures. Weight-bearing exercises, even simple ones like walking or resistance training, can go a long way in improving bone density and reducing the risk of osteoporosis.

Now, how about social interactions? One of the unintended but delightful outcomes of taking fitness seriously is the social aspect. Whether it's a morning walk, or a group exercise class designed for seniors, the opportunities to interact can be a significant mood booster. Isolation can be a substantial issue in senior years, and what better way to combat it than making friends while getting fit?

Ever heard of the term "functional fitness"? It means training your body for the activities performed in daily life. For example, you need lower body strength to climb stairs and upper body strength to carry groceries. Well-rounded fitness routines focus on improving these functional aspects of fitness, making your everyday tasks not just doable but enjoyable.

And let's not forget the cognitive benefits. Regular exercise is not just good for the body; it's also a tonic for the brain. Studies have shown that regular physical activity can enhance cognitive function and delay the onset of conditions like Alzheimer's. So, when you're working out, think of it as a gym session for your brain.

Being fit also offers a sense of accomplishment. Remember, it's never about competing with anyone else; it's about being a better version of yourself. Each day you exercise, you prove to yourself that you can overcome challenges, regardless of age. That alone can be a significant morale booster and a fantastic way to improve self-esteem.

I get it; fitness might seem like a tall order. But it's not about transforming overnight. It's about taking small, consistent steps towards a healthier lifestyle. And the best part? The benefits are almost immediate. From better sleep to improved mood and enhanced physical capabilities, the advantages of maintaining a fit lifestyle as a senior are manifold.

BENEFITS OF RESISTANCE BAND WORKOUTS

"Your body can stand almost anything. It's your mind that you have to convince." —
Unknown.

So, you're sold on exercise and keen on making it a regular part of your life. Fantastic! But why resistance bands? What's the big deal? Well, grab a comfy seat—though not too comfortable because we've got some workouts to do later—and let's chat about the manifold benefits of resistance band workouts.

Resistance bands are like the Swiss Army knife of fitness tools. They're versatile, easy to use, and can be stashed anywhere. But that's just scratching the surface. These stretchy wonders offer a unique form called "linear variable resistance." The more you stretch them, the harder they work against you. This allows for a broad range of motion, giving you a dynamic and comprehensive workout.

Now, about those muscles. Building strength isn't solely about lifting weights or doing push-ups until you drop. Resistance bands offer a unique way to engage multiple muscle groups simultaneously. When you're pulling or pushing against the tension, you're essentially activating different sets of muscles. This gives you a more balanced strength-building approach, unlike traditional weights that often focus on isolated strengths. In simple terms, it's a full-body tune-up in every session.

Indeed, you've heard that consistency is critical, right? Well, resistance bands are champions in the accessibility department. There is no need for an elaborate home gym or a costly membership. You can roll out of bed, grab your bands, and get moving. Convenience is one of the most significant barriers people cite when exercising, and resistance bands bulldoze that barrier like a pro.

What about injury prevention? Oh, you're going to love this. Resistance bands are low impact, meaning they're easy on your joints. If you've had your fair share of aches and pains—welcome to the club!—you'll find resistance band exercises are a great way to stay active without aggravating existing issues. They allow you to control the tension and range of motion, reducing strain or injury risk.

How does this translate to your daily life? Imagine carrying groceries, climbing stairs, or standing up from a seated position. These functional movements rely on strength, balance, and flexibility. The beauty of resistance band workouts is that they prepare you for these everyday activities, making them more accessible and more comfortable to perform.

Elevating your heart rate is another golden ticket; resistance bands can do that, too. While they're not a replacement for cardio, incorporating them into a high-intensity interval training (HIIT) routine can give your heart a good workout. The constant tension from the bands, combined with quick movements, can get your heart pumping just as effectively as a jog around the block.

Mental well-being also gets a boost from resistance band workouts. Physical activity releases endorphins, the body's feel-good hormones. So, not only are you sculpting a more muscular physique, but you're also fostering a more resilient mindset. It's a win-win situation.

And don't forget the cost factor. Resistance bands are budget-friendly, making them a go-to choice for those who want to be mindful of spending without compromising quality. Compared to pricey gym equipment, these bands offer excellent value for their myriad benefits.

SETTING REALISTIC GOALS AND EXPECTATIONS

"A goal without a plan is just a wish." —
Antoine de Saint-Exupéry.

First things first, let's talk about timelines. Setting a deadline creates a sense of urgency and serves as a motivating factor. Think about short-term goals—like being able to do ten leg curls with a light resistance band within two weeks—and long-term goals, like progressing to a medium resistance band within two months.

Why not aim for the stars? Go big or go home, right? Well, slower. Overshooting can lead to disappointment; nothing kills motivation faster than feeling like a failure. So, set goals that stretch your abilities but are still within reach. Nothing boosts confidence like a series of small wins.

Now, you also need to define what success looks like for you. Is it being able to carry your groceries without panting? Or is it about improving your core strength to play with your grandchildren without discomfort? See, every individual's 'finish line' is different. So, decide on yours, and let that be your guiding light throughout this process.

It's also crucial to keep tabs on your progress. Do you know how you meticulously note down recipes or keep records of your favorite books? Yeah, treat your fitness journey with the same level of commitment. Jot down your exercises, resistance levels, and feelings during each session. This not only helps you track your progress but also allows you to make necessary adjustments to your routine.

While we're on the subject of adjustments, be prepared to pivot. Life happens; maybe you'll catch a cold, or a family emergency will pull you away from your routine. That's okay. Don't beat yourself up. Instead, reassess your goals and timelines, make the required adjustments, and keep moving forward.

Another helpful tip is to share your goals with someone you trust. It could be your spouse, a close friend, or even a community of like-minded individuals online. Sharing your objectives makes you more accountable. Plus, a little cheerleading from someone who cares about you never hurts, does it?

Lastly, celebrate your victories, both big and small. Did you complete a full set of exercises that you initially found challenging? That calls for a mini celebration! Reward yourself with something that makes you happy; it could be a favorite meal, a day out doing something you love, or even a new set of exercise clothes.

SAFETY CONSIDERATIONS AND PRECAUTIONS

"Safety doesn't happen by accident." —
Unknown.

First, address the elephant in the room—your exercise environment. Whether it's a corner in your living room or a dedicated home gym, ensure the space is clutter-free. The last thing you want is to trip over a misplaced shoe while in the middle of a leg curl. Keep your workout area clean, well-lit, and ideally, close to something sturdy you can grab onto if you lose your balance.

Now, about those resistance bands. They might look harmless, but if not handled correctly, they can snap, and I assure you, that's not an experience you want to have. Always check your bands for any signs of wear and tear before using them. Tiny cracks or frayed edges signal that the band needs to be replaced. It's better to be safe than sorry, right?

Starting with too much resistance is like jumping into the deep end before you've learned to swim. It's tempting, but trust me, it's a bad idea. Begin with lighter resistance and work up as you become more comfortable, and your muscles get used to the new routine.

Proper technique is another cornerstone of safety. Ever heard of the saying, "It's not about how much you do, but how well you do it"? It rings true here. Incorrect form not only diminishes the effectiveness of the exercise but also increases your risk of injury.

Breathing. It sounds simple enough, but you'd be surprised how many people hold their breath during exercise, especially when it gets challenging. Holding your breath can lead to unnecessary stress on your cardiovascular system. Make sure you're breathing consistently throughout your exercise. A general rule of thumb is to exhale during the exertion phase and inhale during the relaxation phase.

What about attire? Believe it or not, what you wear can impact your safety. Avoid loose, baggy clothing that could get tangled in the bands. Opt for form-fitting, comfortable attire, allowing a full range of motion. Shoes are a bit of a debate in the resistance band community. Some prefer the natural grip of bare feet, while others swear by athletic shoes for better support. The choice is yours, but make sure whatever you choose is slip-resistant.

Hydration is another facet often overlooked. Your muscles are working hard and need adequate hydration to function optimally. A dehydrated body is more susceptible to cramps and fatigue. So, keep that water bottle handy and take sips regularly, even if you don't feel particularly thirsty.

Last but not least, listen to your body. No, listen. Stop immediately if something feels off or you experience unusual pain. It could indicate that you're overexerting yourself or doing an exercise incorrectly. Remember, it's always better to pause and reassess than to push through and regret it later.

COMMON MISTAKES PEOPLE MAKE WHEN USING RESISTANCE BANDS

"Success does not consist in never making mistakes but in never making the same one a second time." - George Bernard Shaw.

This quote rings true regarding using resistance bands for workouts, especially for seniors. Resistance bands are fantastic for building strength, improving flexibility, and enhancing balance. But, like any exercise equipment, they need to be used correctly to avoid injury and get the most out of the workout.

One common mistake is choosing the wrong resistance level. As seniors, it's crucial to start with a lower resistance to protect the joints and muscles. Jumping into a higher resistance band without conditioning the body can lead to unnecessary strain and potential injury. Increasing resistance as strength and endurance build over time gradually is better.

Another mistake is using incorrect forms during exercises. Proper form is critical for safety and ensuring the correct muscles are targeted during each exercise. It's easy to cheat or use momentum rather than muscle power, but this won't bring the desired benefits. Instead, focusing on slow, controlled movements will improve results and help avoid injury.

Not maintaining tension in the band throughout exercises is another issue. The point of resistance training is to keep the muscles under constant tension. If the band slackens during the exercise, the muscles get a break, reducing the workout's effectiveness. Keeping the band taut throughout the movement will ensure the muscles stay engaged and the workout is effective.

Neglecting to control the release of the band can also lead to problems. It's not just the contraction part of the exercise that is important; the release of the 'eccentric' part of the movement is equally crucial. Letting the band snap back quickly doesn't give the muscles the full benefit of the exercise and can also be a safety hazard. Controlling the release ensures a full range of motion and helps build strength and flexibility more effectively.

Overstretching the band is another common mistake. Although resistance bands are flexible, they do have a limit. Stretching the band beyond its capacity can damage the band and increase the risk of it snapping, leading to potential injury. It's essential to use the band within its limits and choose a higher resistance band if necessary.

Ignoring pain or discomfort while using resistance bands is a mistake that can lead to serious injury. It's important to differentiate between a challenging workout's discomfort and a potential injury's pain. If any exercise causes pain, it should be stopped immediately, and a healthcare provider should be consulted before continuing.

The final common mistake is not caring for the bands correctly. Resistance bands are made of latex and can degrade over time, especially if exposed to heat or sunlight. They should be stored in a cool, dry place and checked regularly for signs of wear and tear. Using a damaged band increases the risk of breaking during a workout, which can lead to injury.

TROUBLESHOOTING COMMON ISSUES

In the fitness journey, we face some hurdles. As seniors, it's normal for some workouts not to go as planned. Troubles might pop up now and again. Don't worry. This section aims to help you navigate common problems that might arise while using resistance bands for your exercises.

First, let's talk about discomfort or pain during workouts. If you feel any pain during exercise, stop. Pain is your body's way of telling you something isn't right. Taking a break is okay, and you should never push through the pain. It could indicate improper technique or that the exercise level is too challenging.

Next, let's discuss the issue of balance. Many seniors worry about falling while exercising. To address this, ensure your workout area is clean and free of obstacles. Also, consider exercises you can do seated or lying down until you build up your balance.

Then, let's tackle the problem of feeling too tired. It's common to feel tired when you start a new exercise routine. But if you're feeling exhausted, it might be a sign of overdoing it. Remember, it's okay to start slowly and gradually increase your workout's intensity.

Another common issue is resistance bands snapping or breaking. While rare, it can happen, especially if the bands are old or damaged. Make sure to inspect your resistance bands before each workout. Look for nicks, tears, or any signs of wear and tear.

Some seniors might find it tough to grip the resistance bands. If you're having trouble, consider using resistance bands with handles or wrap the bands around your hands for a better grip.

If you're having trouble feeling the burn during your workouts, it might indicate that you're ready to move up to a higher resistance level. As you get stronger, you must adjust your resistance bands to continue challenging your muscles.

Another common issue is the need for more motivation. It's normal to have days where you don't feel like exercising. When this happens, remind yourself of why you started this journey. Remember, every little bit helps; even a short workout is better than no workout.

Next, let's address the problem of waiting to see results. Remember, progress takes time. Keep going if you see immediate changes. Consistency is key, so stick with it.

INCREASING RESISTANCE AND INTENSITY SAFELY

"Strength does not come from physical capacity. It comes from an indomitable will." - Mahatma Gandhi.

The beauty of resistance band workouts, especially for seniors, is their scalability. You can adjust the intensity and resistance to meet your fitness level. It's not about pushing until it hurts. It's about slowly and steadily increasing the challenge, allowing your body to adapt and grow stronger.

For beginners, it's best to start with a light resistance band. This band offers less resistance, making the exercises easier to perform. It's a great way to introduce your body to new movements and build initial strength. As you progress, you'll notice the exercises becoming more accessible. This is a sign it's time to move up to a medium resistance band.

The medium resistance band is suitable for those at an intermediate fitness level. If you've been exercising regularly and feel comfortable with the movements, this band can add a new challenge to your routines. It offers more excellent resistance than the light band, helping build strength and endurance.

For experienced users, a heavy resistance band is your tool of choice. This band provides the most resistance, demanding more from your muscles. It's a great way to increase the intensity of your workouts, pushing your strength and endurance to new levels. But remember, it's not about the resistance level of the band but how well you can control and perform the movements.

As you progress with your resistance band workouts, remember to be patient. Strength and fitness don't improve overnight. It's a process that requires consistency, patience, and, most importantly, a positive attitude. Remember, it's not about how much you can lift but how well you can lift it.

Incorporating resistance bands into your exercise routine is a safe and effective way to improve your fitness. They're versatile, portable, and can be used anywhere - from your living room to the park. They're perfect for anyone with various resistance levels, regardless of fitness level.

So, pick up a resistance band and start your journey to a stronger, healthier you. Remember, age is just a number. It's always possible to start exercising and improve your quality of life.

Just know that every small step toward your fitness goals makes a big difference. So, keep going, pushing, and, most importantly, believing in yourself. You're stronger than you think.

Chapter 2: Getting Started

CONSULTATION WITH A HEALTHCARE PROFESSIONAL

"Health is a state of complete physical, mental, and social well-being, and not merely the absence of disease or infirmity." — World Health Organization.

You've got the gist of how resistance bands can elevate your workouts, and you're raring to go. You're practically eyeing that set of bands online, finger hovering over the 'Add to Cart' button. But wait a minute! Before diving into this new regimen, one critical step shouldn't be brushed aside: consultation with a healthcare professional.

Yep, it might sound like a bureaucratic roadblock on your path to fitness, but it's more like a green light that ensures you're good to go. Think about it. Your body is as unique as your fingerprint. No two individuals, not even twins, have the same physiological response to exercise. There are always nuances, which are precisely why a healthcare professional's insight can be invaluable.

So, what can you expect from this consultation? Well, for starters, a comprehensive check-up to assess your overall health status. This usually involves blood tests, mobility tests, and perhaps even cardiovascular examinations. You see, even if you feel like a million bucks, there could be underlying conditions you're unaware of. A thorough check-up can flag these potential issues so that you can tailor your exercise regimen accordingly.

Now, let's talk about medication. Many seniors are on some form of drugs for chronic conditions. Whether it's blood pressure, diabetes, or arthritis meds, these can impact how your body reacts to exercise. For example, certain blood pressure medications may affect your heart rate, which could be an essential metric while working out. A healthcare professional will be able to guide you on how to navigate these nuances.

Have pre-existing injuries or mobility issues? Don't sweep them under the rug; bring them to the table during your consultation. A qualified healthcare professional can provide recommendations for exercises that are both safe and effective for your specific condition. Maybe those leg curls you were so eager to try out would put too much strain on your knee joint. In that case, an alternative exercise might be just as effective but far less risky.

And let's not forget the importance of getting the correct form and posture. While resistance bands are generally safe and user-friendly, incorrect usage could lead to muscle strains or even injuries. Your healthcare provider can guide you on the importance of form and may even recommend a few sessions with a physical therapist. These experts can break down each exercise movement, ensuring you're not inadvertently harming yourself in your quest for fitness.

Your dietary habits could also come under the scanner during this consultation. Nutrition and exercise are two sides of the same coin. You can't focus on one and ignore the other. The healthcare professional might ask about your eating habits, suggest some changes, or even recommend visiting a dietitian. Trust me, a little professional guidance on what fuels you can make a world of difference to your workouts and overall well-being.

CARE TIPS, COMMON MISTAKES TO AVOID

"Health is a state of complete physical, mental and social well-being, and not merely the absence of disease or infirmity." - World Health Organization.

When it comes to maintaining our health as seniors, it's essential to understand the proper methods and techniques. Resistance bands are a safe and effective way to keep fit, promote flexibility, and enhance balance. However, like any workout, it's crucial to follow the correct steps and avoid common mistakes that can lead to injury or hinder progress.

The first tip is to be consistent with your resistance band workouts. Consistency is vital in achieving and maintaining our fitness goals. It's about doing a little at a time but making a small effort regularly. Remember, it's a marathon, not a sprint.

Next, pay close attention to your form. Proper form is essential in every exercise to target the intended muscles and prevent injuries effectively. Doing an exercise incorrectly can lead to strain and discomfort. When in doubt, seek guidance from a fitness professional or reputable online resources.

Remember to warm up before starting your workout. Warming up prepares your body for exercise, increasing blood flow and loosening muscles. It can be as simple as a brisk walk or light stretching. Skipping this step can lead to muscle strains or other injuries.

Equally important is cooling down after your workout. This phase allows your body to gradually return to its normal state, reducing the likelihood of muscle soreness and stiffness. Gentle stretching or a slow walk can be an effective cool-down.

Ensure to hydrate. Water is essential for many bodily functions, including maintaining body temperature and lubricating our joints. Drink plenty before, during, and after your workout to prevent dehydration.

Another common mistake is using the wrong resistance band. Resistance bands come in different levels of resistance, from light to heavy. Choose a band that suits your current fitness level. Using a band with too much resistance can strain your muscles and joints.

Check your resistance bands regularly for signs of wear and tear. Over time, they can become worn out and may snap during a workout. Replace them as necessary to prevent accidents.

Take your time with your exercises. Each movement should be controlled and deliberate. Rushing can lead to improper form, reducing the effectiveness of the exercise and increasing the risk of injury.

Avoid holding your breath during exercise. Breathing throughout your workout is essential to supply your muscles with needed oxygen. A good rule of thumb is to exhale on the effort and inhale on the release.

CHOOSING THE RIGHT RESISTANCE BANDS

"The best things in life are often waiting
for you at the exit ramp of your comfort zone." —
Karen Salmansohn.

The market is flooded with options, so how do you narrow it down? For starters, let's talk about the types of resistance bands. You've got tube bands with handles, loop bands, therapy bands, and even figure-eight bands. Each one has its unique features and is best suited for specific exercises. Tube bands, for instance, are great for mimicking gym machine exercises and targeting specific muscle groups. Loop bands, on the other hand, are more for general strength training and physical therapy. What you choose largely depends on the exercise you'll be doing. So, a little bit of pre-planning wouldn't hurt.

Now, let's get into the nitty-gritty—resistance levels. These bands don't play around; they range from light to extra heavy. Lighter bands are typically used for exercises that target smaller muscle groups, like the biceps or triceps. Heavier bands are your go-to for targeting larger muscle groups, like the legs and back. However, starting at a level where you can perform the exercises with good form is crucial. No one's giving out medals for using the heaviest band and throwing out your back. So, start light and work your way up as your strength improves.

Color coding is often used to denote resistance levels, but don't be fooled; there's no universal color scheme. One brand's medium resistance might be another brand's heavy. So, always check the packaging or product details for the resistance level. If you're new to this, consider getting a set with multiple resistance levels. This allows you to mix and match, making your workouts more dynamic and engaging.

Material matters, too. Most resistance bands are made of latex, which offers excellent elasticity and durability. However, if you're allergic to latex, opt for bands made of TPE (thermoplastic elastomer), a non-latex synthetic material. Also, take a moment to inspect the band's width and thickness. A broader and thicker band will generally offer more resistance and is less likely to snap. Trust me; the last thing you want is a snapped band in the middle of a hamstring curl.

If you plan to use your bands for various exercises, look for ones with adjustable handles or attachments. These accessories can add a new dimension to your workouts, allowing for a broader range of movements and grip options. Just think about it: with a door anchor, your living room door suddenly becomes a workout station for tricep pushdowns or lat pulldowns.

So, you've got your type, resistance level, material, and possible accessories sorted. What's next? Before making that purchase, check for user reviews or professional recommendations, especially from sources focusing on senior fitness. These insights can be incredibly helpful in identifying the band's comfort, durability, and effectiveness. After all, you want something that's tried and tested, not a band that will disintegrate after several uses.

PROPER WARM-UP AND COOL-DOWN TECHNIQUES

"To enjoy the glow of good health, you must exercise." — Gene Tunney.

Like revving a car engine on a chilly morning, your body deserves a proper warm-up before you put it through the paces. No, sprinting right out of the gate isn't doing you any favors—unless you're looking to win a one-way ticket to Injuryville. And while we're on the subject, let's not forget the cool-down. Think of it as the "power off" sequence for your body's machinery, helping to ensure that everything winds down smoothly, without any hitches.

Warm-ups prepare your body for the more intensive activity ahead. They get your blood flowing, warm up your muscles, and allow you to prepare for your workout mentally. Imagine jumping right into a high-intensity resistance band exercise; not only would it feel like your muscles were on fire, but the risk of straining something would also skyrocket. A simple warm-up, such as a brisk walk or light cardio for 5–10 minutes, followed by dynamic stretching, can make a difference. Dynamic stretching is the way to go here. We're talking leg swings, arm circles, and torso twists—movements that mimic the exercise you're about to do.

The cool-down is equally important but often overlooked. After a strenuous workout, your heart rate is up, your muscles are tired, and your body has produced waste products like lactic acid. Stopping abruptly can cause blood to pool in your extremities, leading to dizziness or fainting. To avoid this, spend another 5–10 minutes on a light activity like walking. After that, move on to static stretching, where you hold a stretch for 15–30 seconds. This helps increase flexibility, relaxes muscles, and reduces muscle soreness. Static stretches target the muscles you've worked out, so if it's leg day, focus on hamstring, quad, and calf stretches.

What about resistance bands in warm-ups and cool-downs, you ask? Oh, they're more versatile than you might think. For warm-ups, resistance bands can be used for low-resistance, high-rep exercises that target the same muscle groups you plan to work out. For example, if your workout focuses on the upper body, arm circles with a light resistance band can warm your shoulders nicely. For the cool-down, you can use the band for static stretches, elongating the muscles you've just worked out. Picture this: holding one end of the resistance band in your hand and looping the other around your foot to pull it towards you, getting a deep stretch in your hamstring.

But hey, while we're on the subject of proper techniques, posture needs your attention, too. Poor posture during exercise is a leading cause of injuries. So always keep that back straight, shoulders relaxed, and knees slightly bent. It's like the framework that holds up a building; if it's skewed, expect problems.

UNDERSTANDING AND MANAGING JOINT PAIN

"Pain is inevitable. Suffering is optional."
— Haruki Murakami

Ever wake up feeling like you've been hit by a truck, and you know it's those pesky joints acting up again? Joint pain can be a real party pooper. But guess what? It doesn't have to dominate your life. The notion that you're doomed to a life of pain just because you're getting older is outdated. Sure, your joints might not be as spry as in your 20s, but that's no reason to throw in the towel.

So, why do joints even ache? Well, there are a bunch of reasons. Sometimes, it's due to arthritis; other times, it might be an old injury acting up, or it could even be something as simple as overuse. Understanding the root cause is the first step in managing the discomfort effectively. You don't need a medical degree, but chatting with a healthcare provider can offer valuable insights.

Considering you're keen on using resistance bands, you're already ahead of the game. The beauty of resistance bands is their versatility. These handy tools can be adapted to suit various strength levels and target different muscle groups to alleviate or prevent joint pain. For instance, if your knees are troublemakers, leg curls with a resistance band can strengthen the muscles around the knee joint, offering it more support.

And what about those wrists? Ah, so crucial for almost everything, from opening a jar to typing an email. Wrist flexor and extensor exercises using a resistance band can do wonders here. You'll be amazed at how simple movements make everyday tasks much more comfortable.

Of course, exercise isn't the only tool in your arsenal. Did you know that diet plays a significant role in joint health? Omega-3 fatty acids found in fish like salmon are known to reduce inflammation, one of the primary culprits behind joint pain. So, adding a serving or two of fatty fish to your weekly diet can go a long way.

But hold on, we've talked about resistance bands and diet; what about the elephant in the room? Stress. You'd be surprised how much emotional and mental stress can manifest as physical pain. That's why practices like mindfulness and meditation are not to be brushed off as mere new-age mumbo jumbo. They can genuinely help in reducing the stress that exacerbates joint pain.

And when it comes to stress relief, never underestimate the power of a good night's sleep. Sleep is when the body gets a chance to repair and rejuvenate itself. Poor sleep affects your mood and cognitive functions and can interfere with the body's healing ability, making joint pain even more unbearable.

MODIFICATIONS FOR SPECIFIC CONDITIONS

"If you can't fly, then run. If you can't run, then walk. If you can't walk, then crawl, but whatever you do, you have to keep moving forward." — Martin Luther King Jr.

Take arthritis, for instance. It's a condition that can make every joint scream in protest. The natural inclination might be to avoid movement to lessen the pain, but that's where resistance band exercises come in. You can perform a range of joint-friendly movements that help improve flexibility and lessen the severity of arthritis symptoms.

But what if you're dealing with osteoporosis? Ah, the bane of aging bones. While it might seem counterintuitive, strength training is often recommended for managing osteoporosis. The trick is to focus on low-impact, weight-bearing exercises that don't put undue stress on the bones. Resistance band exercises are a fantastic option here. You can perform various exercises that target the hips, spine, and wrists, which are the areas most susceptible to fractures due to osteoporosis.

Have you ever had a sprained ankle or a similar minor injury? It's frustrating, especially when itching to return to your exercise routine. But even here, modifications can save the day. For example, seated resistance band exercises can allow you to keep up with your upper body workouts while giving that sprained ankle the rest it needs.

Now, I get it. Modifying exercises can seem daunting, especially if you're new to the fitness arena. But here's the good news: you don't have to do it alone. Always consult your healthcare provider for personalized advice tailored to your specific condition. They can provide valuable insights into what types of exercises would be most beneficial for you and any modifications that may be necessary.

And then there's the mental aspect. It's easy to feel defeated when dealing with a condition that limits mobility or causes pain. But remember the words of Martin Luther King Jr.: "You have to keep moving forward." When modified to fit your specific condition, exercise can be a powerful tool for physical well-being and mental and emotional wellness.

OVERCOMING BARRIERS TO EXERCISE

"The greatest glory in living lies not in never falling, but in rising every time we fall." —
Nelson Mandela.

The idea that barriers can be steppingstones rather than stumbling blocks isn't new, but it's often easier said than done, right? Especially when it comes to exercise. Maybe you've had days when even putting on your gym shoes felt like climbing Mount Everest. Or perhaps you've wondered if you're too old to start a fitness routine. First, kudos for even pondering these issues because acknowledging them is the first step toward resolution.

So, what are these so-called barriers? Time constraints, physical limitations, and sometimes, let's admit it, a lack of motivation. These obstacles have a funny way of accumulating, turning what should be a simple, health-boosting activity into an ordeal. But here's the kicker: every barrier can be overcome, and often, the solution is simpler than you think.

Time, for instance, is a tricky one. In our heads, exercise often morphs into this monumental task that requires hours of dedication. But who says you need to work out for an hour? Short, focused sessions can be just as practical. Ten minutes of concentrated resistance band exercises can work wonders for your strength and flexibility. Plus, these sessions can easily fit into any schedule. Before breakfast? Sure. During your favorite TV show? Why not?

Physical limitations can be another roadblock. If mobility is a concern, the good news is that many exercises are adaptable. For example, if standing for long periods is uncomfortable, many resistance band exercises can be done while seated. The point is you don't have to fit into the exercise; the exercise can be tailored to fit you.

Now, about motivation. This one's a bit nebulous, isn't it? Some days, you feel like you can conquer the world; others, the couch seems the most attractive option. The key here is to find your "why." Why do you want to exercise? Is it to keep up with your grandkids? To maintain your independence? Or perhaps to manage a health condition? Identifying your underlying motivation can be the fuel you need to get moving, even on days when inertia sets in.

But what if you stumble? What if you miss a day, a week, or a month? Well, remember Mandela's words: "The greatest glory in living lies not in never falling, but in rising every time we fall." If you've fallen off the exercise wagon, the best time to return is now. Not tomorrow, not the following Monday—now. And if you're worried about starting all over, don't be. Muscle memory is beautiful; your body will remember, and you'll return to your old routines quicker than you think.

Chapter 3: Boosting Balance and Stability

THE NEED FOR BALANCE

"Life is a balance of holding on and letting go." — Rumi

What Rumi, the 13th-century Persian poet, captured in a single sentence speaks volumes about the human condition. Balance isn't just a metaphorical concept; it's a physical reality, especially as we age. We often underestimate how much a simple task, like picking up a fallen newspaper, relies on our body's ability to maintain equilibrium. A slight mishap, like tripping over a shoe, can instantly transform from a minor inconvenience to a significant ordeal. That's why balance, my friend, is more than a buzzword; it's a cornerstone of your well-being.

So, why all this fuss about balance? Well, for starters, it's not just about preventing falls, but that's a crucial part. Balance aids in every movement, from walking to reaching for a can on the top shelf. That intangible quality keeps you steady, confident, and safe in your movements. You see, balance is intricately tied to your muscle strength and flexibility. You become this harmonious blend of capability and agility when these elements align. You're not just moving; you're moving with purpose and control.

It gets better. Improved balance doesn't just keep you upright; it enhances your overall quality of life. Think about it. When you trust your body to be stable, you're more likely to engage in activities that bring joy and meaning. Whether gardening, playing with your grandkids, or simply taking a leisurely walk in the park, balance paves the way for a fuller, more active life.

But let's be clear. Balance isn't a given; it's a skill. Like any skill, it requires regular practice and mindful attention. Thankfully, the human body is an adaptable machine. Even if you've spent years neglecting this aspect of your health, it's never too late to make amends. A bit of focused effort can yield impressive results. That's the beauty of our physiology; it's eager to reward us when we invest in it.

BEGINNER EXERCISES

"Take care of your body. It's the only place you have to live." — Jim Rohn.

The journey to building strength, balance, and flexibility begins with simple steps. For seniors, these steps include easy-to-follow exercises designed to cater to their needs. Using resistance bands, these exercises can be performed at home, offering a convenient way to enhance physical well-being.

SEATED ROW

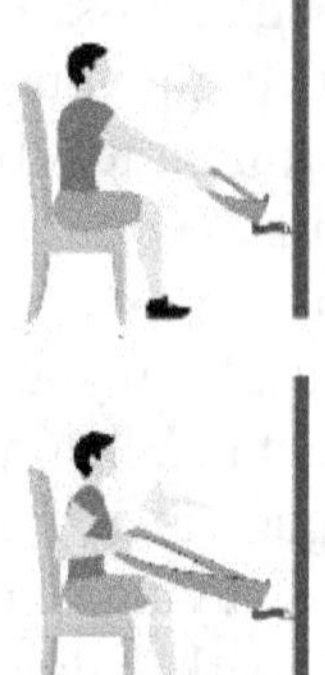

The Seated Row exercise focuses on strengthening the upper body, particularly the back and shoulder muscles. Here's how to do it:

1. Sit on a chair and keep your feet flat on the floor.

2. Attach a resistance band to a sturdy object at chest level.

3. Hold the ends of the band with your arms straight out in front of you.

4. Pull the band towards your body until your elbows are by your sides.

5. Slowly extend your arms back to the starting position.

6. Repeat for 15 reps.

LEG PRESS

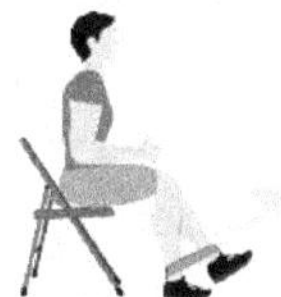

The Leg Press exercise improves lower body strength. Here's how to perform it:

1. Sit on a chair with your feet flat on the floor.

2. Place a resistance band around your ankles.

3. Extend one leg forward, keeping the other foot stationary.

4. Slowly bring your leg back to the starting position.

5. Repeat with the other leg.

6. Do this for ten reps per leg.

CHEST PRESS

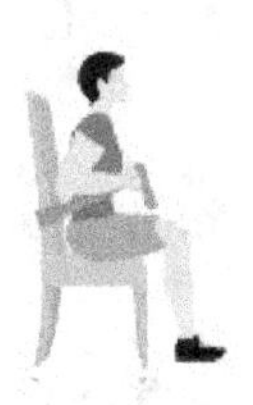

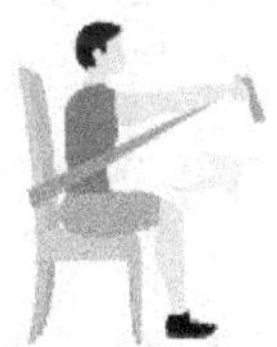

The Chest Press exercise targets the chest and arm muscles. Here's how to do it:

1. Sit on a chair with your feet flat on the floor.

2. Wrap a resistance band around your back, holding the ends with each hand.

3. Push your arms forward, extending them fully.

4. Slowly return to the starting position.

5. Repeat for 15 reps.

BAND PULL-APART

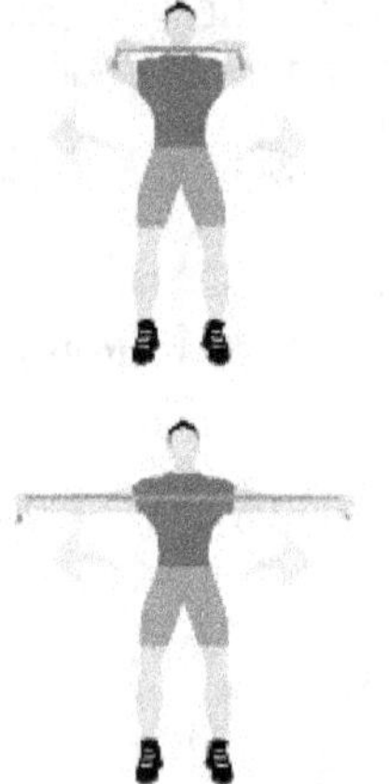

BAND PULL-APART

The Band Pull-Apart is a practical upper back and shoulder exercise. Here's how to perform it:

1. Stand with your feet shoulder-width apart.

2. Hold the resistance band in front of you with both hands, arms fully extended.

3. Without bending your elbows, pull the band apart by squeezing your shoulder blades together.

4. Slowly return to the starting position.

5. Repeat for 15 reps.

BICEP CURL

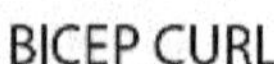

BICEP CURL

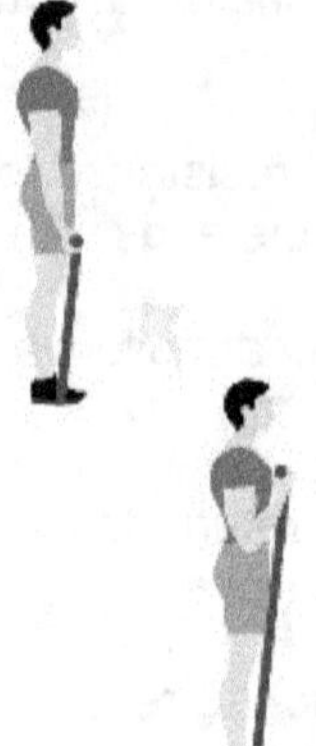

The Bicep Curl exercise strengthens arm muscles. Here's how to do it:

1. Stand in the middle of the resistance band, holding the ends with each hand.

2. Keep your elbows close to your body and palms facing forward.

3. Curl your hands towards your shoulders, keeping your elbows stable.

4. Slowly lower your hands back to the starting position.

5. Repeat for 15 reps.

EXERCISES FOR IMPROVING CORE STRENGTH FOR BETTER BALANCE

The essence of balance lies in the core. A strong core is vital for stability, mobility, and overall strength. And for seniors, this becomes even more crucial. Fear not, as you can build this strength right at home with resistance bands. Here are five exercises designed to help you do just that.

SEATED RUSSIAN TWIST

SEATED RUSSIAN TWIST

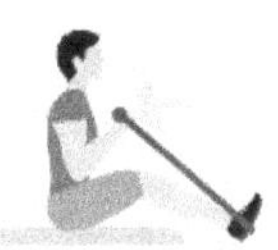

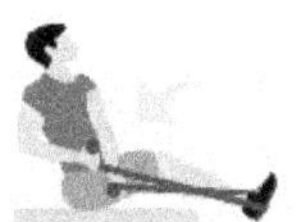

The Seated Russian Twist is an effective core exercise that targets your oblique muscles.

1. Sit on the floor with your knees bent and feet flat.

2. Hold the ends of the resistance band with both hands, arms fully extended in front of you.

3. Slowly rotate your torso to the right, then to the left, to complete one rep.

4. Do this for about 10 to 15 reps.

BAND BICYCLE CRUNCH

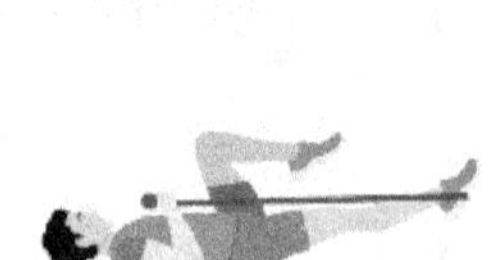

The Band Bicycle Crunch helps engage your lower abs and obliques.

1. Lie flat on your back, legs extended, and hold the band handles with both hands.

2. Bend your left knee and bring it towards your chest while moving your right elbow towards it.

3. Return to the starting position and repeat on the other side for one rep.

4. Perform 10 to 15 reps per side.

BAND PUSH-DOWN

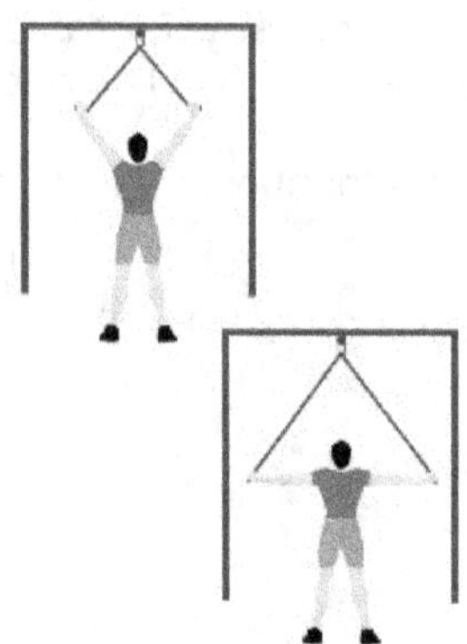

The Band Push-Down is a great way to engage your core while targeting your upper body.

1. Stand with your feet hip-width apart.

2. Hold the resistance band in both hands, arms fully extended above your head.

3. Push your arms down, engaging your core until they are at your sides.

4. Slowly raise your arms back up to the starting position.

5. Repeat for 10 to 15 reps.

BAND SIDE BEND

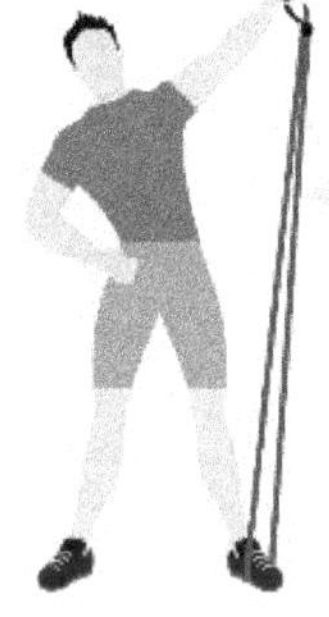

The Band Side Bend is a simple but effective exercise for your obliques.

1. Stand with your feet hip-width apart, holding the band in your right hand.

2. Extend your right arm overhead, keeping your elbow close to your ear.

3. Bend to the left, engaging your right oblique.

4. Return to the starting position and repeat for 10 to 15 reps.

5. Switch sides and repeat.

BAND WOOD CHOP

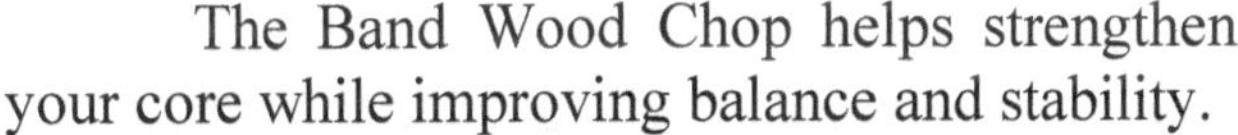

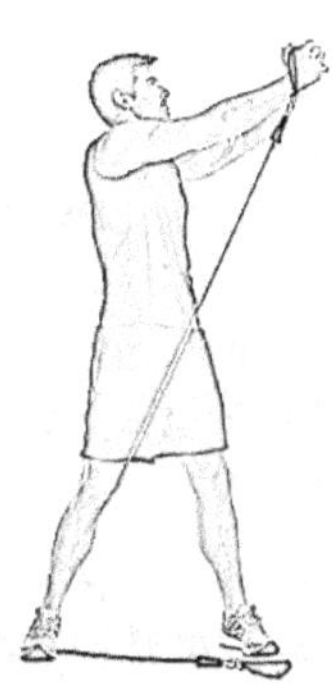

The Band Wood Chop helps strengthen your core while improving balance and stability.

1. Stand with your feet shoulder-width apart, holding the band in both hands.

2. Rotate your torso to the right, extending your arms diagonally up to the right.

3. Then, in a chopping motion, pull the band diagonally across your body to your left knee.

4. Return to the start position to complete one rep.

5. Do this for about 10 to 15 reps on each side.

EXERCISES FOR ENHANCING COORDINATION AND PROPRIOCEPTION

"Wellness is not a 'medical fix' but a way of living—a lifestyle sensitive and responsive to all the dimensions of body, mind, and spirit, an approach to life we each design to achieve our highest potential for well-being now and forever."—Greg Anderson.

Every senior citizen deserves a life full of vibrancy, strength, and balance. One way to achieve this is through exercises that enhance coordination and proprioception. Let's dive into five accessible, safe, and highly effective exercises.

LATERAL BAND WALKS

The Lateral Band Walks are intended to strengthen your hips and glutes, which are crucial for maintaining balance.

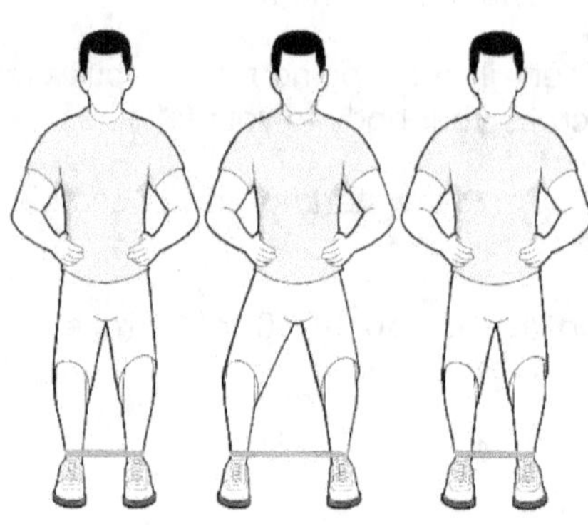

1. Stand with your feet hip-width apart. Place the resistance band around your ankles.

2. Keep your hands on your hips or extend them in front of you for balance.

3. Step to the right with your right foot, then follow with your left foot.

4. Continue for ten steps, then repeat in the opposite direction.

SQUATS WITH BAND

Squats with Bands are perfect for strengthening your lower body and improving your balance.

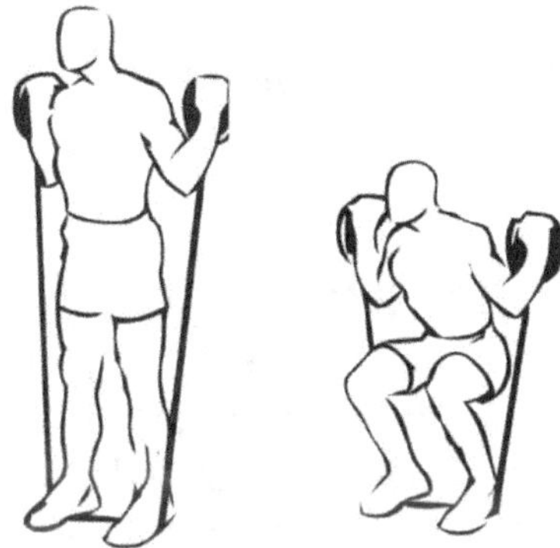

1. Stand on the resistance band with feet shoulder-width apart. Hold the band with both hands at shoulder level.

2. Squat down as if sitting on a chair, keeping your chest lifted.

3. Push back up to standing and repeat for 15 reps.

SEATED LEG EXTENSION

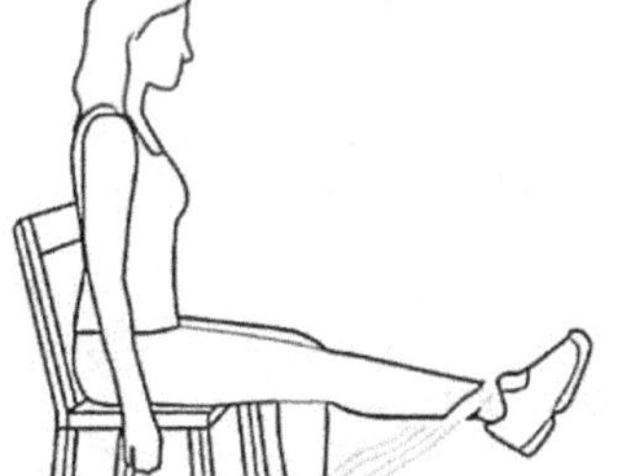

Seated Leg Extension targets the quadriceps, a crucial muscle group for maintaining leg balance and strength.

1. Sit on a chair with the resistance band looped around your ankles.

2. Extend one leg before you, then slowly bring it back down.

3. Repeat for 15 reps, then switch to the other leg.

TARGETED EXERCISES FOR FALL PREVENTION

"The resistance that you fight physically in the gym, and the resistance that you fight in life can only build a strong character." - Arnold Schwarzenegger.

Let's dive into five targeted exercises for fall prevention. They're designed to help you enhance your balance, strength, and overall well-being. I've handpicked these exercises to tackle limited mobility and poor balance. They are easy to perform at home, using resistance bands.

SIDE LEG LIFTS

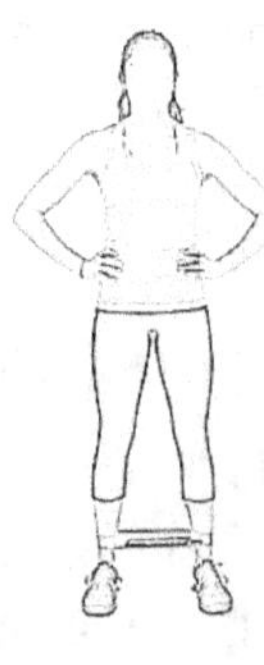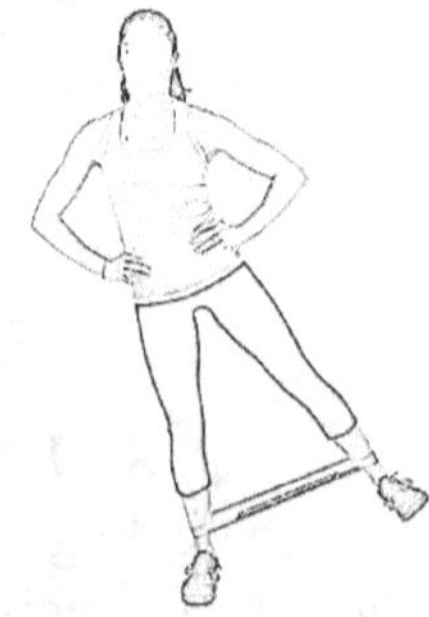

Side Leg Lifts engage your hip and thigh muscles. This workout is simple but effective.

1. Stand with your feet hip-width apart.

2. Place the resistance band around your ankles.

3. Lift your right leg to the side, keeping your body straight.

4. Slowly lower your right leg.

5. Repeat with your left leg for one rep.

6. Do this for 15 reps.

FRONT LEG RAISES

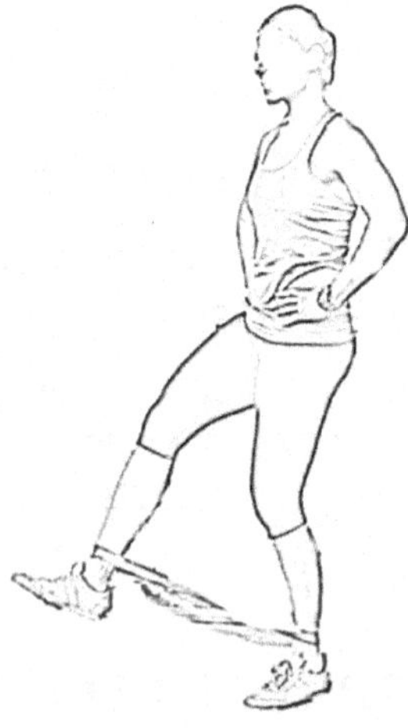

Front Leg Raises target your thigh and hip muscles. This exercise is both easy and impactful.

1. Stand with your feet hip-width apart.

2. Put the resistance band around your ankles.

3. Lift your right leg before you without bending your knee.

4. Slowly lower your right leg.

5. Repeat with your left leg for one rep.

6. Do this for 15 reps.

CHAIR SQUATS

Chair Squats engage your lower body muscles. This workout is simple yet valuable.

1. Stand in front of a chair with your feet hip-width apart.

2. Loop the band around your thighs just above your knees.

3. Bend your knees and lower your body as if sitting down.

4. Push back up to the starting position.

5. Repeat for 15 reps.

OVERHEAD PRESS

The Overhead Press works out your shoulder and arm muscles. This exercise is straightforward but significant.

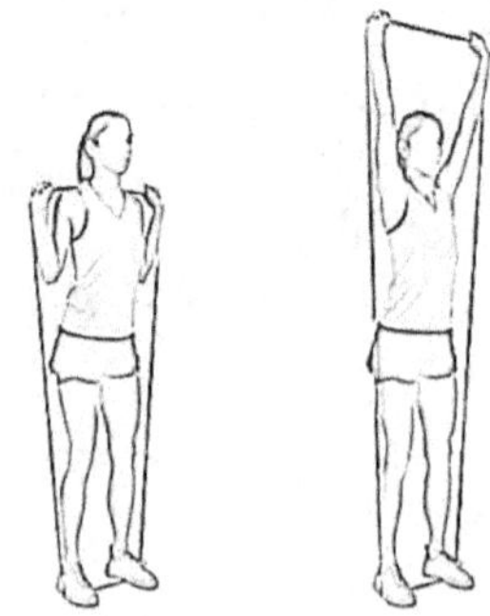

1. Sit or stand with your feet hip-width apart.

2. Hold the band at shoulder height with your palms facing forward.

3. Push your hands up and extend your arms.

4. Lower your hands back to shoulder height.

5.   Repeat for 15 reps.

STRETCHING AND FLEXIBILITY EXERCISES

"The resistance band is a simple yet profound tool. It's like having a whole gym in your hand." - Unknown.

We dive into five stretching and flexibility exercises. Each exercise uses resistance bands. We'll detail the level of resistance needed for beginners, intermediates, and experienced users.

DOORWAY CHEST STRETCH

The Doorway Chest Stretch opens up your chest and shoulders. It's great for correcting posture and relieving tension.

1. Secure a band in a door jam at chest height.

2. Stand facing the door and hold the ends of the band with your arms extended to the sides.

3. Gently lean forward until you feel a stretch in your chest.

4.   Hold for a few seconds, then return to the starting position.

5.   Repeat for 15 reps.

BAND-ASSISTED HAMSTRING STRETCH

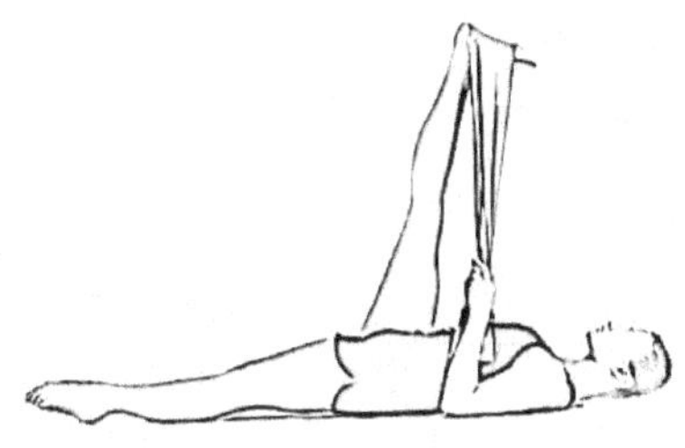

The Band-Assisted Hamstring Stretch relieves tension in your hamstrings and lower back.

1. Lie flat on your back with your legs extended.

2. Loop a band around one foot and hold the ends in both hands.

3. Lift your leg and gently pull the band towards you until you feel a stretch in your hamstring.

4. Hold for a few seconds, then return to the starting position.

5. Repeat for 15 reps on each leg.

STANDING CALF STRETCH

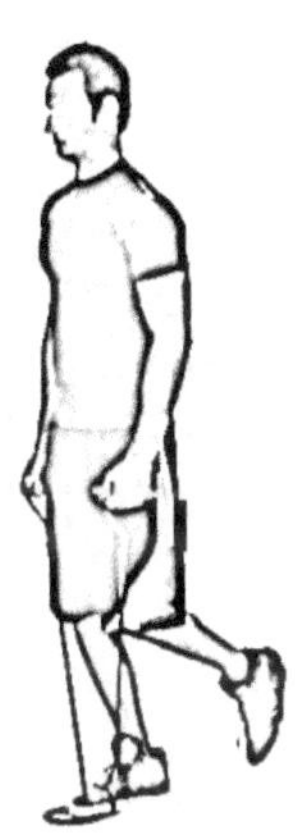

The Standing Calf Stretch targets your calf muscles. It's ideal for enhancing lower body flexibility.

1. Stand facing a wall with a band looped around one foot.

2. Hold the other end of the band with your hands.

3. Pull the band towards you while keeping your heel on the ground.

4. Hold for a few seconds, then return to the starting position.

5. Repeat for 15 reps on each leg.

SEATED LOWER BACK STRETCH

The Seated Lower Back Stretch relieves lower back tension and improves flexibility.

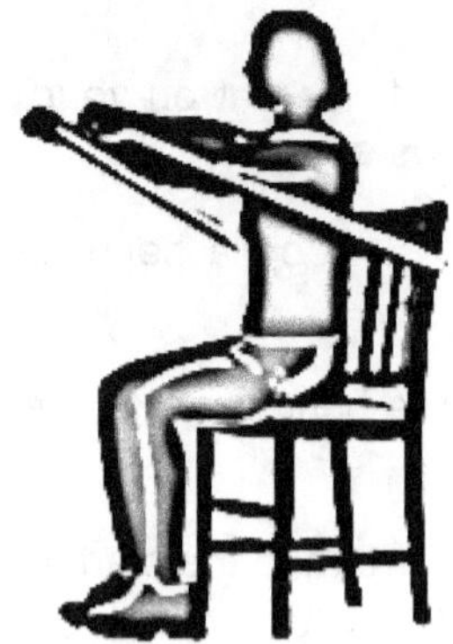

1. Sit on the edge of a chair with your feet flat on the floor.

2. Hold a band with both hands, arms extended in front of you.

3. Lean forward from your hips, resisting the band's pull.

4. Hold for a few seconds, then return to the starting position.

5. Repeat for 15 reps.

EXERCISES TO ALLEVIATE BACK AND NECK PAIN

"Amid movement and chaos, keep stillness inside of you." - Deepak Chopra.

Managing back and neck pain can be challenging, especially for seniors. However, incorporating resistance band exercises into your routine can help you manage these discomforts effectively. These affordable, convenient, and versatile exercises allow you to work out different muscle groups with a single tool.

OVERHEAD BAND STRETCH

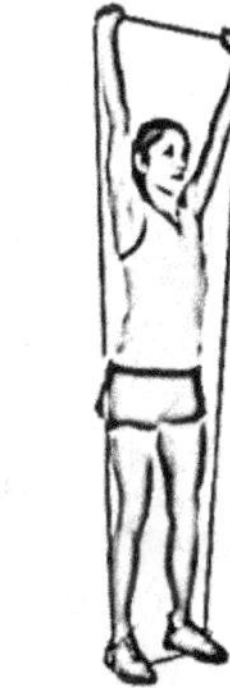

The Overhead Band Stretch is a gentle exercise that helps in relieving neck pain and tension.

1. Sit or stand upright.

2. Hold the resistance band slightly wider than shoulder-width apart with both hands.

3. Slowly raise your arms over your head, stretching the band.

4. Lower your arms back down.

5.	Repeat this motion for 15 reps.

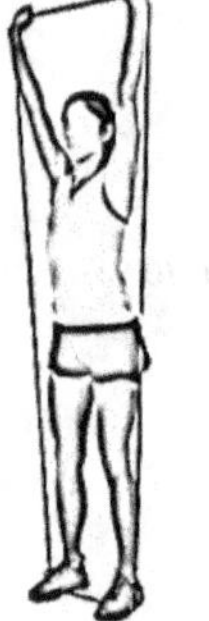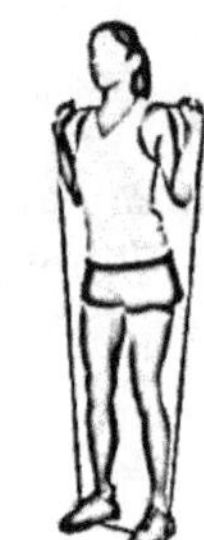

RESISTANCE BAND PULL DOWN

The Resistance Band Pull Down exercise strengthens the upper back and neck muscles.

1.   Stand upright and hold the band over your head.

2.   Pull the band down while bending your elbows.

3.   At the end of the movement, your elbows should be at your sides.

4.   Slowly raise your arms back to the starting position.

5.   Repeat this for 15 reps.

BAND-ASSISTED NECK STRETCH

Band Type: Light resistance band for beginners, medium for intermediate, and heavy for experienced.

The Band-Assisted Neck Stretch is a gentle exercise to relieve tension and stiffness in the neck.

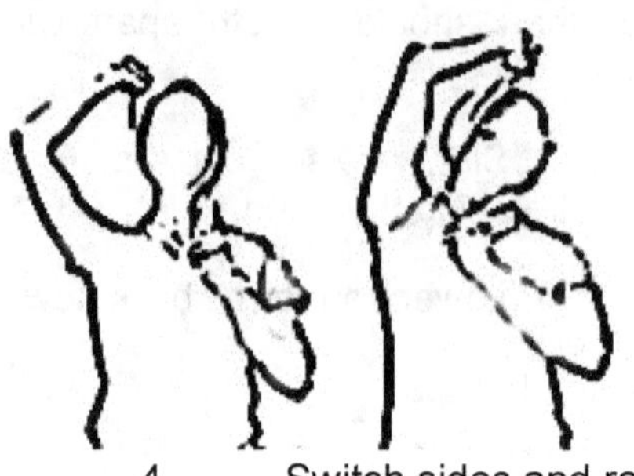

1. Sit upright on a chair.

2. Hold one end of the band in your right hand and the other end draped over your left shoulder.

3. Gently pull the band to the right side, stretching the left side of your neck.

4.   Switch sides and repeat.

5.   Do this for ten reps on each side.

SHOULDER SHRUG

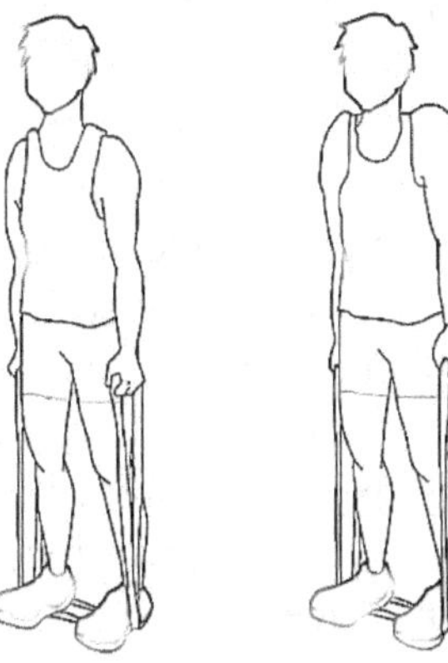

The Shoulder Shrug is a simple yet effective exercise to alleviate shoulder and neck pain.

1. Stand on the resistance band.

2. Hold the ends of the band in each hand.

3. Shrug your shoulders up towards your ears.

4. Slowly lower your shoulders back down.

5.	Repeat for 15 reps.

INCORPORATING BALANCE EXERCISES INTO EVERYDAY ACTIVITIES

"Life is like riding a bicycle. To keep your balance, you must keep moving." - Albert Einstein.

The key to a vibrant life isn't necessarily found in drastic changes or elaborate routines. Sometimes, the secret sauce to improving your well-being hides in the mundane, everyday activities you already do. That's right, your daily life is chock-full of opportunities to enhance your balance and, by extension, your overall health. You don't need an Olympic-size swimming pool or a deluxe home gym to make a difference. The living room, the kitchen, and even the bathroom offers a stage for you to perform little acts of balance.

Why should you care about balance exercises? Imagine the body as a finely tuned machine; the system might fail if one-part malfunctions. Balance, my friend, is the unsung hero that keeps you upright and functional. It plays a pivotal role in nearly everything you do, from walking to standing up from a chair to bending over to tie your shoelaces. Yet, it's something many people take for granted—until they struggle to maintain it. So, let's fix that, shall we?

Remember brushing your teeth this morning? Turn that into a mini-balance exercise by standing on one leg. Sounds too simple? Sometimes, simplicity is the real genius. Not only are you making those leg muscles work, but you're also enhancing proprioception—the body's ability to sense its location in space. It's like killing two birds with one stone, except you're not killing anything; you're giving life to your muscles and balance.

Cooking dinner? Use the counter for support and practice leg lifts or ankle rolls while waiting for that pot to boil. These small, almost inconsequential movements can improve stability and prevent falls. The kitchen counter is not just a space for culinary art; it's also your new fitness buddy.

Have you ever found yourself waiting for the microwave to ding or the coffee to brew? That's a prime time to practice your toe stands or heel lifts. Lift your heels off the floor, stand on your tiptoes, and lower yourself back down. A couple of reps here and there, and you'll find your calf muscles and sense of balance thanking you in the long run.

Walking from room to room? Why not throw in a high-knee march? Raise one knee as high as it will go and then do the same with the other. It might seem silly initially, but these tiny tweaks in your daily routine accumulate significant health benefits. Plus, who's watching? The furniture has seen you do weirder things.

Even watching TV can become a balance-boosting activity. During commercials or a particularly dull scene, why not stand up and do a couple of side leg lifts? Or if you've got a wall nearby, try a wall sit. It's less about the exercise itself and more about seizing the opportunities to make balance a daily habit.

Exercise needs to be this grand, planned event requiring specific clothing, equipment, and a motivational playlist. While that's one way to do it, embedding small exercises into your daily routine can be just as effective, if not more so. The best part? You don't have to carve out extra time from your day. These little "exercise hacks" fit seamlessly into your life, almost as if they were always meant to be there.

Chapter 4: Strengthening Muscles for Better Posture and Mobility

THE IMPORTANCE OF MUSCLE STRENGTH

"Strength does not come from physical capacity. It comes from an indomitable will." - Mahatma Gandhi.

Muscle strength isn't just for bodybuilders or athletes; it's the secret sauce that keeps everyone, including seniors, living their best lives. Who doesn't want the ability to lift their grandkids, carry groceries, or even just rise from a chair without wincing in discomfort? Muscle strength isn't about aesthetics; it's about functionality and freedom.

So why is muscle strength such a big deal, especially as we age? You see, life has a funny way of throwing curveballs at us. One day, you're hiking up a mountain; the next, you struggle to pick up a dropped pen from the floor. It's not a gradual decline; it's often a series of subtle nudges from your body saying, "Hey, we've got to talk." Muscles lose their size and strength, a natural process known as sarcopenia. This decline is sneaky; you might not notice it until you rely on the handrail to climb stairs.

Muscle strength is intricately linked to your ability to perform everyday tasks. Think about how many times you use your muscles in a day. From getting out of bed to opening a jar of pickles, your muscles are always at work. The stronger they are, the easier these tasks become, and the less strain you put on your body. A solid foundation of muscle strength can also protect your joints from injury. Strong muscles act like a built-in shock absorber, taking the brunt of the force when you accidentally trip over a rug.

Now, let's bust a myth: the one that says strength training is all about lifting heavy weights and grunting loudly in a gym filled with sweaty, muscular folks. Nope, not true. Strength training can be incredibly adaptable and suited to your individual needs, especially with resistance bands. These versatile tools can provide a full-body workout that targets every major muscle group, all from the comfort of your home. What's not to love?

Or consider the Standing Leg Curl, an excellent choice for strengthening the hamstrings and glutes. Just tie a resistance band around your ankles, stand straight, and curl one leg at a time towards your glutes. This move is especially beneficial for improving stability and balance, which are crucial as you age.

And don't forget about your core! Yes, those muscles that keep you upright and take the load off your back. Exercises like the Resistance Band Russian Twist can target your core muscles effectively. All you need is to sit on the floor, hold a resistance band with both hands and rotate your torso from side to side. Not only does this strengthen your core, but it also improves your rotational mobility.

Muscle strength is also an unsung hero when it comes to metabolic health. A well-muscled body burns more calories at rest than a body with less muscle mass. This means you can indulge in that extra slice of pie without worrying too much about weight gain, not that I'm encouraging poor dietary choices!

Lastly, let's talk about the psychological benefits. A substantial body often leads to a strong mind. The sense of accomplishment that comes from being able to perform tasks that once seemed challenging can give your self-esteem a significant boost. You become less dependent on others, fostering an invaluable sense of independence, especially when society often unjustly equates aging with dependency.

AGE AND POSTURE CHANGE

"Posture is the outward expression of your inner health. The better you are inside, the better your posture will be." - Jean Couch.

Have you ever caught a glimpse of yourself in the mirror or a window and thought, "Whoa, when did I start slouching like that?" It's a question that often pops up with age, and it's about time we addressed it. Your posture isn't just about how you stand or sit; it's an all-encompassing reflection of your physical health, muscle strength, and emotional well-being. And guess what? Aging has its say in how your posture evolves—or devolves, for that matter.

As the years go by, various factors start influencing your posture. Muscle mass starts to decline, joints stiffen, and your body's natural alignment might get a tad whack. It's almost like your body is subtly rebelling, reminding you that the clock's ticking. But don't let that discourage you. It's never too late to improve your posture and, by extension, your quality of life.

First, let's talk about what age does to your back, the backbone of your posture—pun intended! As you age, the spinal discs, those shock-absorbing cushions between your vertebrae, tend to lose their moisture content. Yep, they dry out. Imagine a juicy, plump grape turning into a raisin. The outcome? A compressed spine and, quite often, a stooped appearance. You may also experience a loss in bone density, making your skeleton more fragile and less supportive of a good posture.

But all isn't lost. Just because you've got a few more candles on your birthday cake doesn't mean you should throw in the towel. Far from it! With the right kind of exercise, you can make a U-turn. Think of resistance bands as your trusty sidekick in this endeavor. Not only are they easy to use, but they're also incredibly effective in targeting specific muscles responsible for a solid, upright posture.

Take, for example, the Pallof Press. This is a fantastic exercise for enhancing core stability. Why does that matter, you ask? Because a strong core serves as the axis around which your entire body functions. When your core muscles are robust, they help maintain spinal alignment, improving your posture.

Then, there's the Banded Pull-down. Picture this as a less-intimidating version of the lat pulldown machine you might find in a gym. This exercise engages your latissimus dorsi, the broadest muscle in your back. Strengthening these muscles will naturally pull your shoulders back, opening your chest and promoting a more upright posture.

The beauty of resistance bands is that they offer an adjustable level of difficulty. As you progress, you can switch to bands with higher resistance, continually challenging your muscles and preventing plateaus. The best part? These exercises are low impact, making them ideal for seniors who may be concerned about joint health.

One might think, "I've been slouching for years; what difference will it make now?" Here's my rebuttal: A lot. Improving your posture can lead to many benefits you might not have considered. We're talking about reduced back pain, improved digestion, and even a boost in confidence. Yes, standing tall makes you feel as good as you look.

THE ROLE OF RESISTANCE BANDS IN POSTURE IMPROVEMENT

*"Your posture is the foundation for every
movement your body makes and can determine
how well your body adapts to the stresses on it." -
Murdoc Knight.*

You know how we often talk about the core? Your body's physical core and your wellness's symbolic core. Well, posture is a cornerstone in that discussion. Good posture isn't just about standing tall for the camera; it's the essential framework that supports your overall health and well-being. And here's the kicker: Resistance bands, those unassuming stretchy loops, can play a pivotal role in enhancing your posture.

First, let's acknowledge that posture is more than a straight back. It's a complex interplay of muscle strength, flexibility, and daily habits. A hunched back, rounded shoulders or a tilted neck doesn't just emerge overnight. These are the results of continuous neglect of your posture, sometimes accentuated by long hours of sitting, perhaps at a desk job, or other lifestyle factors.

Resistance bands are an excellent tool for targeted posture improvement exercises. These bands provide a range of resistance levels, allowing you to challenge multiple muscle groups critical for maintaining a healthy posture. You can effectively counteract the gravitational pull that often leads to a reclined position by focusing on exercises that strengthen your back, shoulders, and core.

Then there's the good old Squat to Press. While you may consider it more of a leg exercise, it's an integrated movement that engages your core and stabilizes your spine, promoting a balanced posture. The key lies in executing these exercises with mindful engagement. You're not just going through the motions; you're actively focusing on the muscles working, creating a mind-muscle connection essential for postural improvement.

For seniors, resistance band exercises have the added benefit of being low impact, meaning they are gentle on the joints. So, whether you're dealing with arthritis or other age-related issues, you can safely use resistance bands to improve posture without exacerbating existing conditions. It's a win-win situation; you enhance your posture and simultaneously work on strengthening various muscle groups, all while keeping things accessible on the joints.

And here's something to chew on: Improved posture doesn't just make you look taller and more confident; it has a domino effect on your health. A well-aligned spine promotes better circulation, efficient digestion, and improved mental clarity. Yes, standing tall is not just a physical state but also a state of mind.

FULL-BODY RESISTANCE BAND WORKOUTS

"Physical fitness is not only one of the most important keys to a healthy body, it is the basis of dynamic and creative intellectual activity." - John F. Kennedy.

In the comfort of your own home, you can engage in a full-body workout using resistance bands. For a comprehensive workout, let's explore five resistance band exercises that activate different muscle groups.

SQUAT TO OVERHEAD PRESS

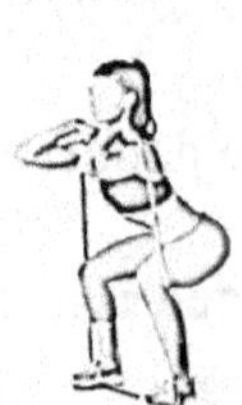
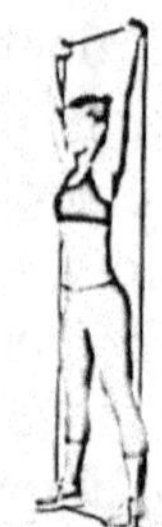

The Squat to Overhead Press is a fantastic exercise that works your lower body and shoulders. It involves a squat and an overhead press, thus engaging multiple muscle groups simultaneously.

1. Stand on the resistance band with feet hip-width apart.

2. Hold the ends of the band at shoulder level with palms facing forward.

3. Perform a squat by bending your knees and pushing your hips back.

4. As you stand back up, press your arms straight up overhead.

5. Lower your arms back to shoulder level as you return to the squat position.

6.   Repeat for 15 reps.

STANDING CHEST PRESS

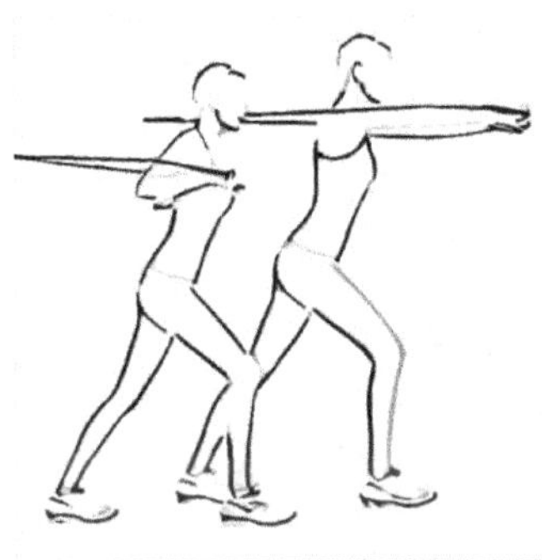

The Standing Chest Press is an effective exercise that targets the chest and triceps.

1. Stand with your back to a post or door and loop the band around it at chest level.

2. Hold the ends of the band at chest level with your elbows bent and palms facing down.

3. Push the band straight out before you, extending your arms.

4.   Bend your elbows to return to the starting position.

5.   Repeat for 15 reps.

EXERCISES FOR BUILDING UPPER BODY STRENGTH

"Strength does not come from winning. Your struggles develop your strengths. When you go through hardships and decide not to surrender, that is strength." - Arnold Schwarzenegger.

In the pursuit of a healthier lifestyle, strength plays a crucial role. When we speak of strength, we often think of the upper body. This section offers five exercises using resistance bands to help build your upper body strength.

SHOULDER PRESS

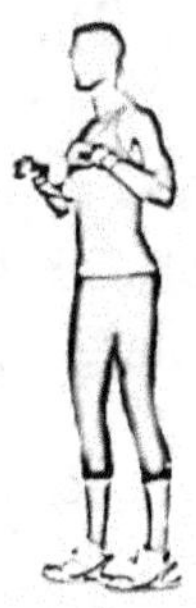
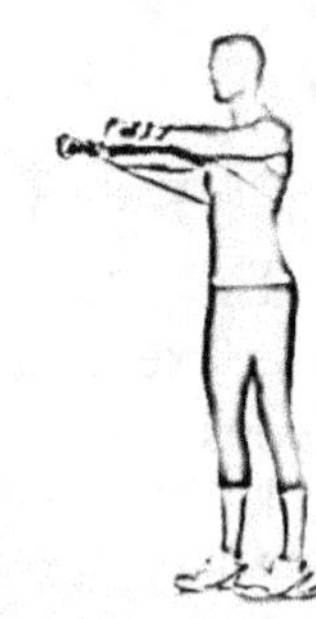

The Shoulder Press is an excellent exercise for enhancing shoulder strength and stability.

1. Stand on the band and hold the ends with your hands at shoulder level.

2. Push your hands upward, extending your arms.

3.   Slowly return to the starting position.

4.   Repeat for 15 reps.

LAT PULL DOWN

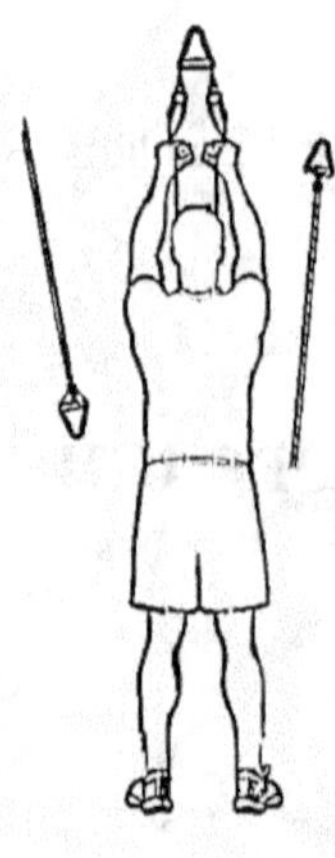

The lat pulldown targets your latissimus dorsi or "lats," a large back muscle contributing to upper body strength.

1.   Secure the band to a high anchor.

2.   Grasp the band with both hands, arms extended.

3.   Pull the band down to your chest.

4.   Slowly return to the starting position.

5.   Repeat for 15 reps.

EXERCISES FOR DEVELOPING LOWER BODY STRENGTH

"Strength does not come from physical capacity. It comes from an indomitable will." -
Mahatma Gandhi.

The essence of lower body strength lies in its impact on our daily lives. It aids seniors in maintaining balance, flexibility, and overall well-being. Resistance band exercises are a great way to build this strength. They are simple, easily adjustable for different fitness levels, and can be done at home. Here, we present five practical lower-body exercises using resistance bands.

BAND GLUTE BRIDGE

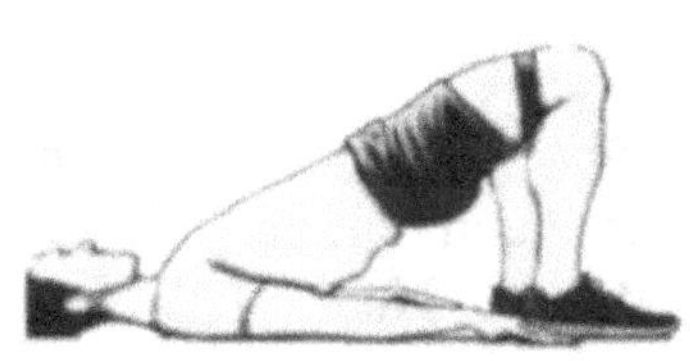

The Band Glute Bridge is a powerful exercise that targets your glutes and hamstrings. It improves your lower body strength and stability.

1. Lie on your back with your knees bent.

2. Place the resistance band around your thighs, just above your knees.

3. Lift your hips off the floor, squeezing your glutes at the top.

4. Slowly lower your hips back to the floor.

5. Repeat for 15 reps.

BAND HAMSTRING CURL

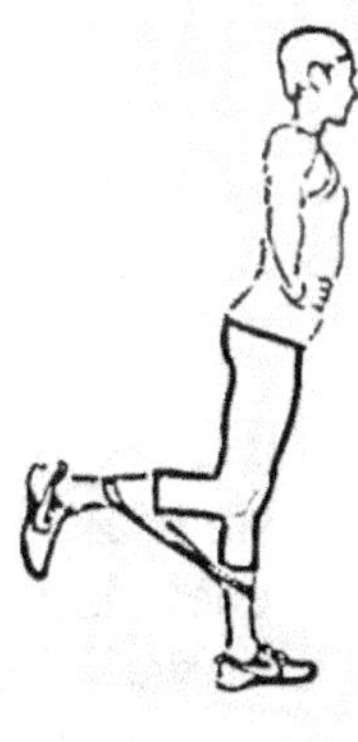

The Band Hamstring Curl is an effective exercise to strengthen your hamstrings. It will enhance your balance and improve your lower body strength.

1. Stand with your feet shoulder-width apart.

2. Place the resistance band around your ankles.

3. Curl one leg back, pulling against the band.

4. Slowly return to the starting position.

5. Repeat for 15 reps on each leg.

Exercises for Strengthening Core Muscles

"The body achieves what the mind believes." - Napoleon Hill

This quote speaks volumes about the power of our mindset regarding physical fitness. The mind and body work together to achieve the desired physical fitness. Now, let's talk about strengthening core muscles using resistance bands.

Resistance Band Bridge

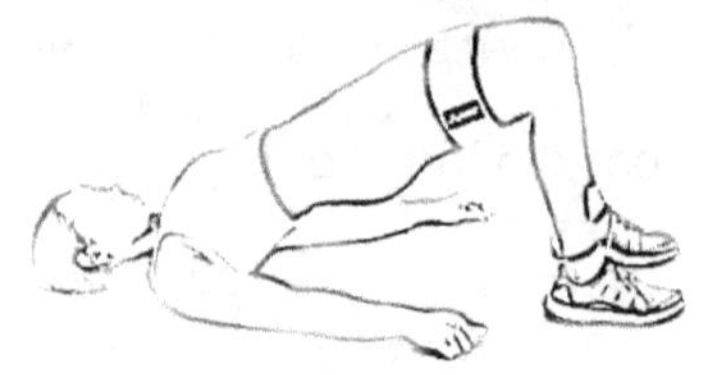

This exercise targets the glutes and hamstrings, which are essential parts of your core. Here's how to do it:

1. Lie on your back with your feet flat on the ground and knees bent.

2. Loop the band just above your knees.

3. Push your hips up while keeping your feet apart against the band's resistance.

4. Lower your hips and repeat 15 times.

Resistance Band Plank

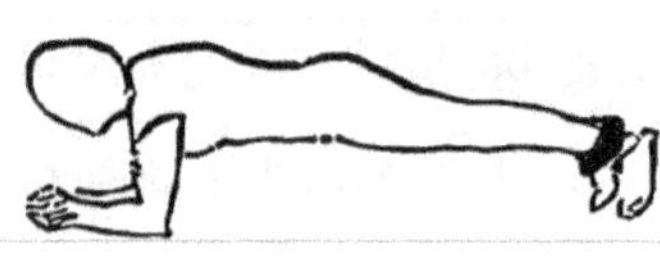

The plank exercise is well-known for its effectiveness in building a solid core. In this variation, the resistance band increases the challenge.

1.   Get into a high plank position with the band around your ankles.

2.   Maintain a straight body line as you separate your feet against the band's resistance.

3.   Bring your feet back together and repeat for 12 reps.

RESISTANCE BAND DEAD BUG

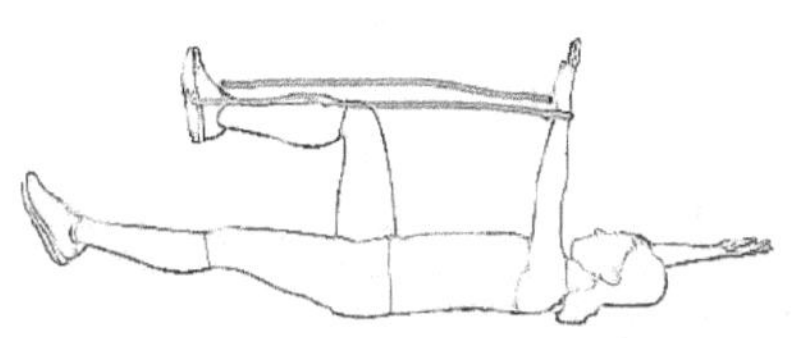

The Dead Bug aims to improve core stability and control.

1. Lie on your back with your arms extended straight up.

2. Loop the band around your feet and hold the ends with your hands.

3.   Extend one leg and the opposite arm, resisting against the band.

4.   Return to the starting position and switch sides. Do ten reps on each side.

DYNAMIC EXERCISES FOR STRONGER BACK AND POSTURE

"Strength does not come from winning.
Your struggles develop your strengths." - Arnold
Schwarzenegger

The body's natural strength may decrease with age, but regular exercise and resistance band workouts can reclaim your power, stability, and posture.

Let's dive into the five dynamic exercises designed to help you regain strength and improve your posture.

STRAIGHT-ARM PULLDOWN

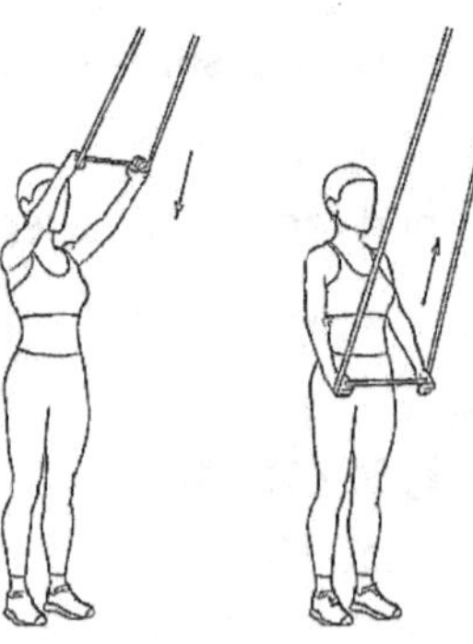

The Straight-Arm Pulldown is a great exercise that targets your latissimus dorsi, the most significant muscle in your back. This workout helps in maintaining a good posture and enhancing upper body strength.

1. Stand upright and anchor your resistance band overhead.

2. Grasp the band with both hands, keeping your arms straight.

3. Pull down the band towards your thighs, keeping your arms straight.

4. Slowly return to the starting position.

5. Repeat for 15 reps.

STANDING BACK EXTENSION

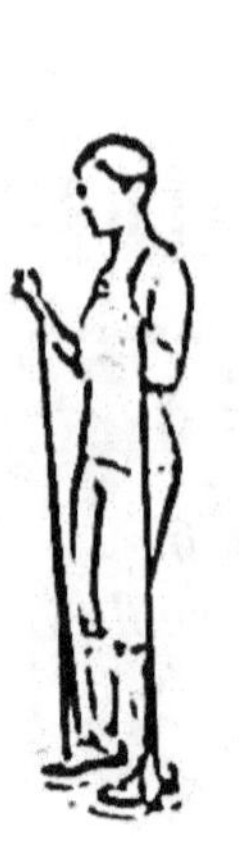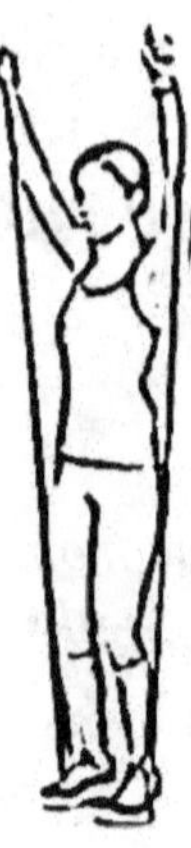

The Standing Back Extension is a fantastic exercise that targets the lower back muscles, improving strength and posture.

1. Stand upright and step on the band.

2. Hold the ends of the band with both hands.

3. Extend your back, pulling the band up with straight arms.

4. Slowly return to the starting position.

5. Repeat for 15 reps.

RESISTANCE BAND DEADLIFT

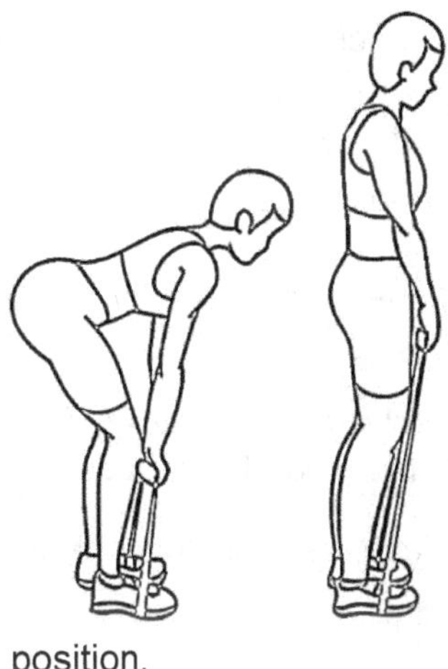

The Resistance Band Deadlift is an excellent exercise that targets the entire back, glutes, and hamstrings, improving overall strength and posture.

1. Stand on the band with feet hip-width apart.

2. Bend at the waist and grasp the band with both hands.

3. Stand up straight, extending your back and legs, pulling the band upward.

4. Slowly return to the starting position.

5.   Repeat for 15 reps.

When performed regularly, these dynamic exercises can significantly improve your back strength and posture. The key, as always, is consistency. Remember that the journey to better health and improved physical strength is a marathon, not a sprint.

EXERCISES FOR CORRECTING ROUNDED SHOULDERS AND FORWARD HEAD POSTURE

Rounded shoulders and forward head posture have become common issues among seniors. These postural problems can lead to discomfort and even pain. But the good news is you can improve your posture and alleviate these issues with the right exercises.

FACE PULL

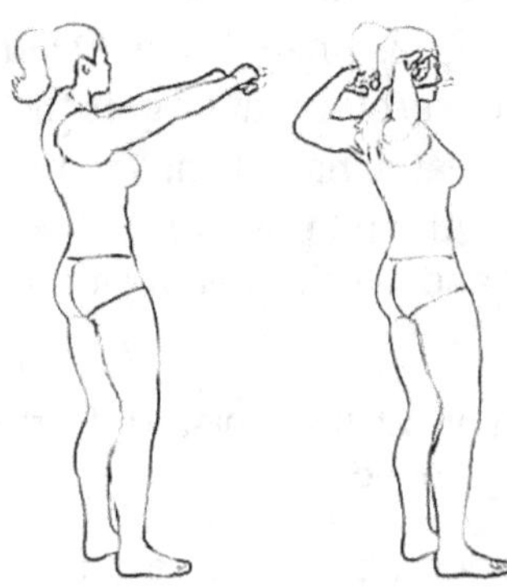

The Face Pull is a fantastic exercise targeting the upper back and neck muscles. It helps in correcting rounded shoulders and forward head posture.

1. Tie the resistance band to a sturdy post at eye level.

2. Stand a few feet away, facing the post, and grasp the band with both hands.

3.   Pull the band towards your face, keeping your elbows high.

4.   Slowly return to the starting position.

5.   Repeat for 15 reps.

OVERHEAD PULL DOWN

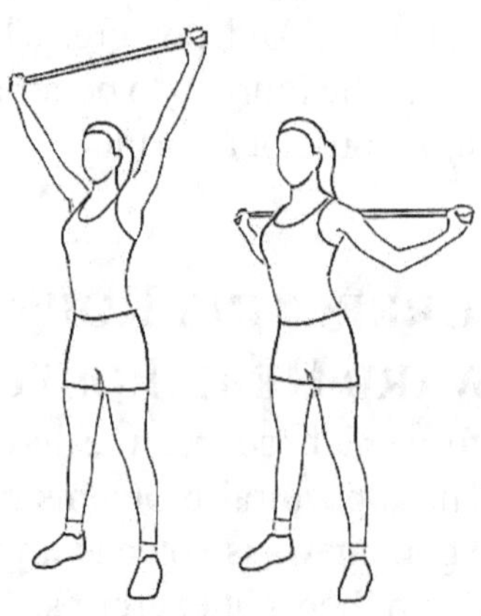

The Overhead pull-down is a simple yet effective exercise to strengthen your upper back and improve your posture.

1. Stand with your feet hip-width apart.

2. Hold the resistance band overhead with both hands.

3. Pull the band behind your head, squeezing your shoulder blades together.

4. Slowly return to the starting position.

5.   Repeat for 15 reps.

WALL ANGELS

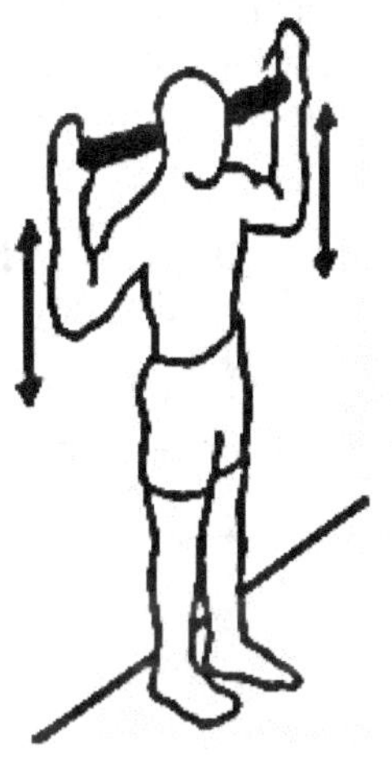

The Wall Angels exercise helps to correct rounded shoulders and forward head posture by targeting the muscles in your back and shoulders.

1. Stand with your back against a wall.

2. Hold the band in front of you with your arms at a 90-degree angle.

3. Slowly raise your arms above your head, keeping contact with the wall.

4. Lower your arms back to the starting position.

5. Repeat for 15 reps.

EXERCISES FOR PROMOTING SPINAL HEALTH AND MOBILITY

Our spine is a pillar of our body, a critical component of our mobility, and pivotal for our overall health. Resistance band exercises are a practical approach for seniors to maintain their spinal health.

BAND-ASSISTED BACK EXTENSION

This exercise strengthens your core, lower back and improves posture.

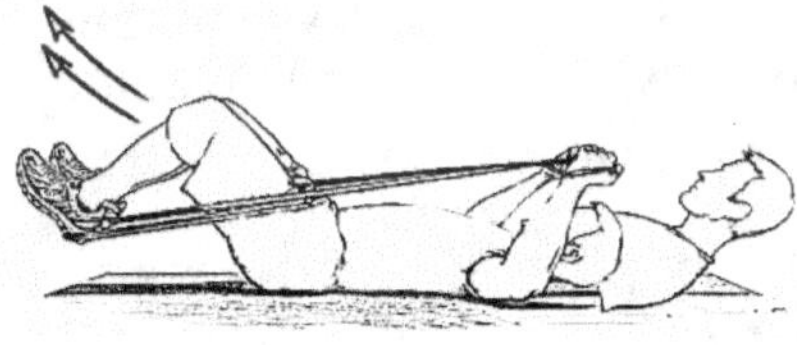

1. Lie face up with the band looped around your feet and hold the ends with your hands.

2. Lift your chest and feet off the floor, pulling the band towards your shoulders.

3. Lower your chest back to the floor.

4. Repeat for 15 reps.

STANDING BAND GOOD MORNING

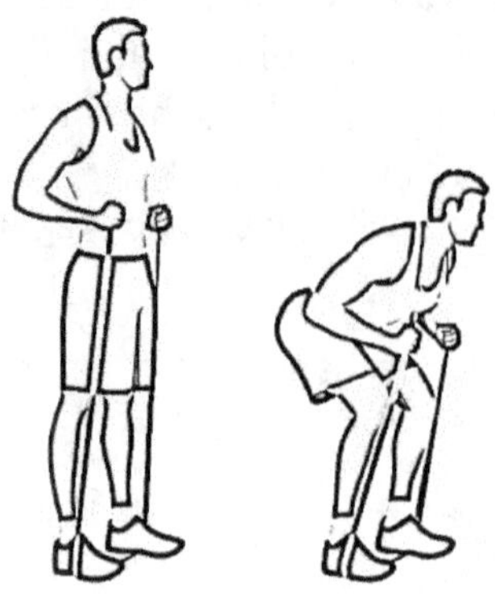

It strengthens the lower back and stretches the hamstrings.

1. Stand on the band with your feet hip-width apart and hold the ends at your shoulders.

2. Maintain a slight bend in your knees and hinge forward from the hips, keeping your back straight.

3. Return to the standing position.

4. Repeat 15 times.

CHALLENGING YOURSELF: PROGRESSIVE OVERLOAD

"Progress is impossible without change, and those who cannot change their minds cannot change anything." - George Bernard Shaw.

How does reaching that plateau in your exercise routine feel? It's like hitting a wall made of marshmallows: soft enough to cushion you but sticky enough to hold you back. For anyone there, progressive overload is the equivalent of a jetpack strapped to your back, propelling you over that wall. Forget what you've heard about staying in your comfort zone; that's where dreams go to die.

In the workout sphere, it's easy to become complacent. You find an exercise routine you're comfortable with and stick to it. You can do the moves; they don't exhaust you to the point of collapse. But ask yourself this: Are you still seeing improvements? If you're shaking your head, don't worry; you're not alone. Stagnation is the enemy of progress, and it's not just you—it's the biology of the human body. We adapt. We adjust. We get comfortable. And comfort is the enemy of growth.

So, what is progressive overload? Think of it as the GPS guiding you through the fitness plateaus and stagnation labyrinth. It's about systematically increasing the stress you put on your body during exercise. You can't expect to build strength, endurance, and flexibility by doing the same old routines at the same old intensities. No, you must challenge your muscles, cardiovascular system, and mental fortitude.

Now, don't get the wrong idea. Progressive overload doesn't mean you should suddenly double the weight you lift or run twice as far. That's a ticket to Injuryville, a place no one wants to visit. Instead, you tweak your workouts in small but impactful ways. Maybe you can add another set of resistance band squats or hold that yoga pose for a few seconds longer. Whatever it is, the change should be enough to make your body sit up and take notice but not so much that it sends you into overexertion.

What's that? Are you wondering who I am to preach this philosophy? Look, I've been in the trenches—literally and figuratively. I've worked with seniors who thought their days of making physical improvements were long gone. But guess what? With the right approach to progressive overload, they made gains that left their jaws on the floor. I know the power of this principle because I've seen it in action and felt it in my own life.

Resistance bands are a godsend for implementing progressive overload, especially for seniors. These versatile tools can be used to add resistance to a variety of exercises. For example, you've been doing seated leg lifts with a light band. After a week, switch to a medium resistance band. It's a small change that sends ripples through your muscles, signaling them to grow stronger.

You may ask, "Isn't it risky for seniors to keep pushing the envelope?" Let me be clear: Progressive overload is not about pushing to the point of pain or extreme discomfort. It's about embracing a bit of struggle in the pursuit of improvement. There's a difference between good pain (muscle fatigue, the burn you feel during exercise) and bad pain (sharp, stabbing sensations or pain that persists). Knowing that difference is crucial.

It's also essential to keep tabs on your body's response. If you notice that your muscles are sore after stepping up your routine, that's generally a good sign. It means your muscles are adapting, repairing, and growing stronger. However, if you experience joint pain or extreme fatigue, it may mean you've pushed too far too fast. In that case, it's perfectly okay to scale back a bit.

Boredom: doing the same exercises day in and day out can be mind-numbingly dull. Progressive overload can be a savior here, too. It not only keeps your muscles guessing but also keeps your mind engaged.

You see, progressive overload is not just a physical concept; it's a mental one, too. It's about pushing your boundaries, not just in terms of muscle and stamina but also mental grit and self-belief. The truth is that the body achieves what the mind believes. If you think you can't, you won't. But if you believe you can, the places you'll go!

Alright, let's get down to the brass tacks. How do you implement progressive overload in your resistance band exercises? Here's a quick rundown: First, start by increasing your resistance band's weight or adding an extra set to your existing routine. Second, make sure you're maintaining proper form throughout your exercises. It's easy to get sloppy when pushing yourself, but poor form can lead to injuries. Third, always give yourself time to rest and recover. Progressive overload is effective only when you allow your body the time it needs to repair and grow stronger.

Remember, implementing progressive overload doesn't mean you'll see results overnight. It's a gradual process but one that guarantees long-term gains. Think of it as investing in a high-interest savings account; the returns may not be immediate but compound over time.

Is progressive overload a silver bullet? No, it's not. But it's a highly effective strategy for breaking through plateaus and continually improving your fitness, regardless of age. And that, my friend, is how you keep the marshmallow walls at bay and soar into a life of ever-improving physical fitness.

Chapter 5: Total Body Workouts with Resistance Bands

STANDING ROW

The Standing Row is a back-strengthening exercise that works your shoulders and biceps.

1. Stand on the band with feet hip-width apart.

2. Hold the ends of the band in each hand.

3. Bend your elbows and pull your hands towards your chest.

4. Extend your arms back to the starting position.

5. Do this for 12-15 reps.

EXERCISES FOR HIGH-INTENSITY INTERVAL TRAINING (HIIT) WITH RESISTANCE BANDS

Resistance band training is a game-changer. It's a simple yet effective way to get a full-body workout. Today, we're focusing on five exercises for high-intensity interval training (HIIT) with resistance bands.

BANDED PUSH-UPS

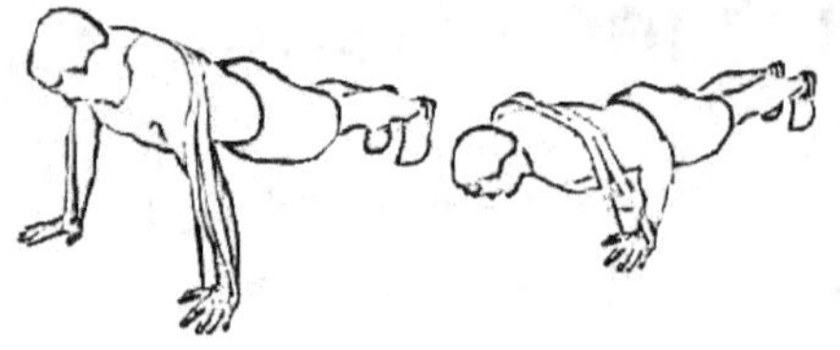

Banded Push-ups add an extra challenge to regular push-ups, working your chest, arms, and core.

1. Get into a high plank position with the band around your back, holding the ends under your hands.

2.   Lower your body, bending your elbows.

3.   Push back to the starting position.

4.   Repeat for 20 seconds, rest for 10, and continue for 4 minutes.

RESISTANCE BAND ROW

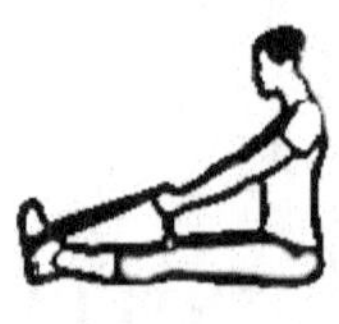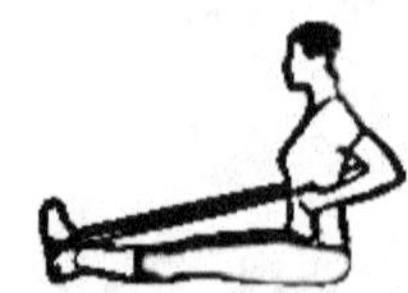

Resistance Band Rows work your back and improve posture.

1. Sit on the floor with your legs extended.

2. Place the band around your feet and hold the ends.

3.   Pull the band toward your waist.

4.   Release slowly.

5.   Repeat for 20 seconds, rest for 10 seconds, and continue for 4 minutes.

CHAIR-BASED RESISTANCE BAND WORKOUT ROUTINE

"Physical fitness is not only one of the most important keys to a healthy body, it is the basis of dynamic and creative intellectual activity." - John F. Kennedy.

Here we are. We'll go through five chair-based resistance band exercises. They're made for seniors in mind. Remember to choose the band that suits your fitness level.

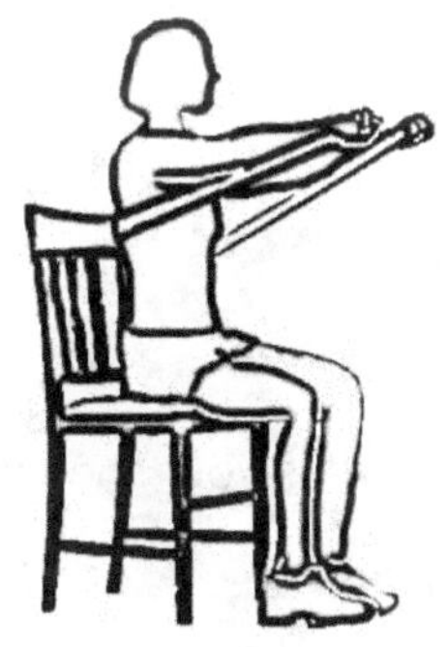

SEATED CHEST PRESS

The Seated Chest Press targets your chest muscles. It's easy but effective.

1. Sit on the edge of a chair.

2. Wrap the band around your back.

3. Hold the ends of the band.

4. Push your hands forward.

5. Slowly bring them back.

6. Repeat for 15 reps.

SEATED LEG PRESS

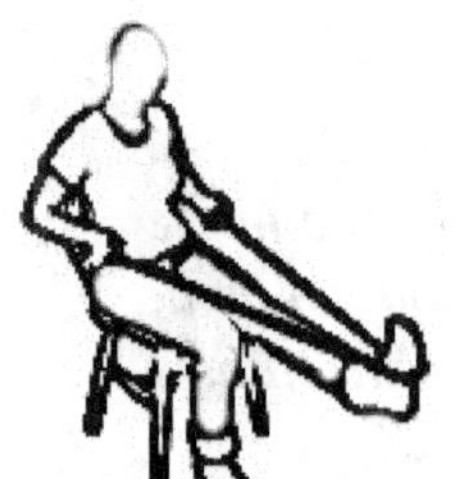

The Seated Leg Press works on your lower body. It's basic but packs a punch.

1. Sit on a chair.

2. Wrap the band around one foot.

3. Hold the ends of the band.

4. Extend your leg.

5.   Slowly return to start.

6.   Repeat for 15 reps.

SEATED BICEP CURL

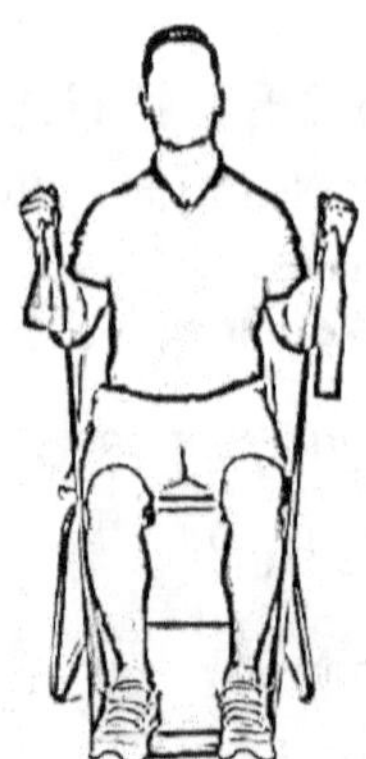

The Seated Bicep Curl helps you tone your arms. It's simple but delivers.

1. Sit on a chair.

2. Step on the band.

3. Hold the ends of the band.

4. Curl your hands towards your shoulders.

5. Slowly lower them down.

6. Repeat for 15 reps.

SEATED OVERHEAD PRESS

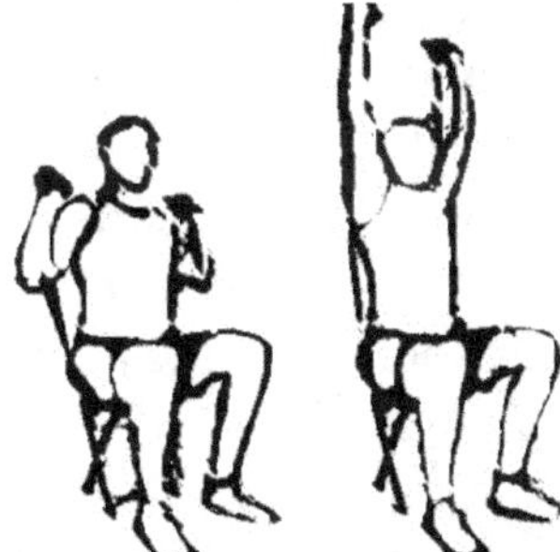

The Seated Overhead Press works on your shoulder muscles. It's easy but does wonders.

1. Sit on a chair.

2. Place the band under your chair.

3. Hold the ends of the band.

4. Push your hands upwards.

5. Slowly bring them down.

6. Repeat for 15 reps.

YOGA-INSPIRED RESISTANCE BAND MOVEMENTS

"Yoga is the dance of every cell with the music of every breath that creates inner serenity and harmony." - Debasish Mridha.

Yoga is not just about flexibility; it's a path for holistic wellness. Today, we'll blend the tranquility of yoga with the strength of resistance bands. Let's learn five yoga-inspired exercises using resistance bands.

RESISTANCE BAND WARRIOR POSE

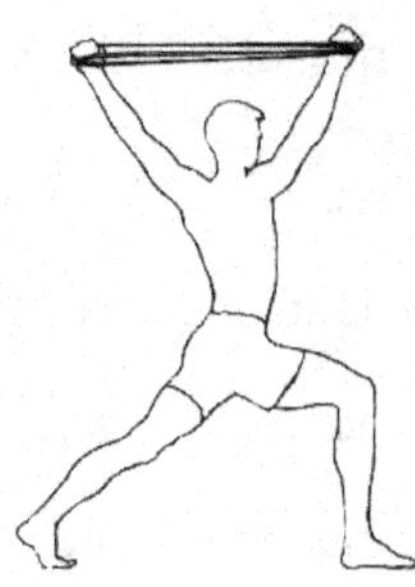

The Resistance Band Warrior Pose is a fantastic method to build lower body strength and improve balance. This pose increases the flexibility of your hips and strengthens your thighs.

1. Stand with your feet wide apart.

2. Turn your right foot out 90 degrees and your left foot in by about 15 degrees.

3. Hold the resistance band with both hands and raise it above your head while bending your right knee.

4. Ensure your right knee is directly above the right ankle.

5. Hold this pose for a few breaths, then switch sides.

RESISTANCE BAND TREE POSE

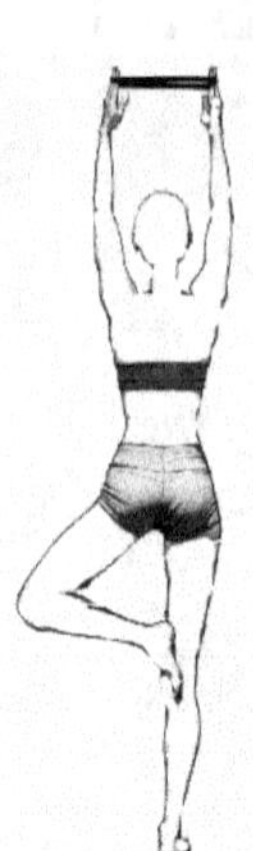

The Resistance Band Tree Pose improves balance and stability, which is essential for our daily activities.

1. Stand tall and shift your weight on the right foot.

2. Bend your left knee and place the sole of your left foot on your right inner thigh.

3. Hold the resistance band with both hands and raise it above your head.

4. Stay in this position briefly, then switch sides.

RESISTANCE BAND CHAIR POSE

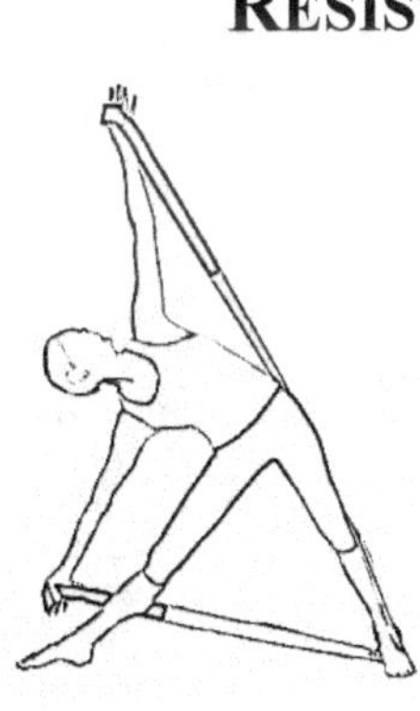

The Resistance Band Chair Pose targets the muscles of your arms and legs. It also strengthens your core and lower back.

1. Start with your feet hip-width apart.

2. Bend your knees as if you are sitting in a chair.

3. Hold the resistance band with both hands and raise it above your head.

4. Stay in this pose briefly, then return to standing.

RESISTANCE BAND BOAT POSE

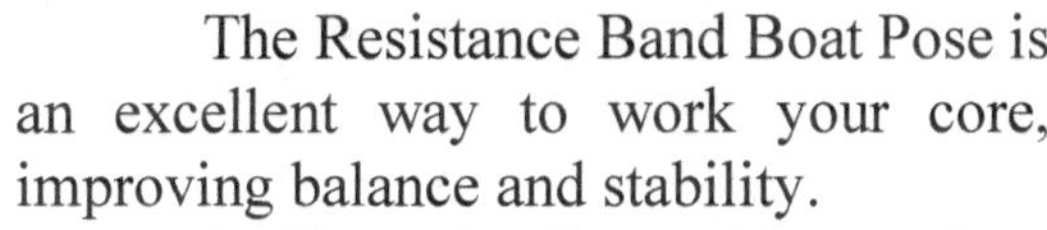

The Resistance Band Boat Pose is an excellent way to work your core, improving balance and stability.

1. Sit on the floor with your legs straight before you.

2. Lean back slightly and lift your feet off the floor.

3. Hold the resistance band with both hands and stretch it over your legs while keeping your balance.

4. Hold this pose for a few breaths, then release.

RESISTANCE BAND TRIANGLE POSE

The Resistance Band Triangle Pose is a great way to stretch your sides and strengthen your legs.

1. Stand with your feet wide apart.

2. Turn your right foot out 90 degrees and your left foot in slightly.

3. Stretch your arms out to the sides.

4. Reach forward with your right hand and touch your right shin.

5. Hold the resistance band in your left hand and stretch it towards the ceiling.

6. Hold this pose for a few breaths, then switch sides.

Chapter 6: Cardiovascular Health and Endurance

The heart is a powerhouse in our bodies. It keeps us going. But as we age, it needs extra care. One way to do this is through resistance band workouts. They are not just for muscle tone and strength. They can help your heart, too.

MANAGING BREATHLESSNESS AND EXERTION

This quote underscores the essence of our topic here: managing breathlessness and exertion.

As we age, the body's capacity to take in oxygen diminishes, making us prone to shortness of breath during physical activities. This can pose a significant challenge, particularly in seniors who wish to maintain an active lifestyle. However, with the right approach, you can control breathlessness and manage exertion effectively while exercising.

INCORPORATING AEROBIC EXERCISES INTO DAILY ROUTINE

"Physical fitness is not only one of the most important keys to a healthy body, it is the basis of dynamic and creative intellectual activity." - John F. Kennedy.

Incorporating aerobic exercises into your daily routine can be a game-changer. It's about making minor, manageable tweaks to your lifestyle. You don't need to spend long hours in a gym. With resistance bands, you can practice effective workouts right at home.

One of the simplest ways to incorporate exercise into your day is to swap sedentary activities with active ones. For instance, you can perform resistance band exercises while watching TV. This approach makes exercise a part of your lifestyle rather than a chore.

It's also beneficial to create a schedule. Consistency is critical when trying to make any lifestyle change. Schedule your workout sessions as you would any other important task. This way, you're more likely to stick to them.

You can also make aerobic exercises a social activity. Working out with a friend or family member can make the whole experience more enjoyable. You can motivate each other and make the sessions more interactive and fun.

Chapter 7: Fine-Tuning Your Routine

"The secret of change is to focus all of your energy, not on fighting the old, but on building the new." - Socrates.

In the realm of fitness, change is the only constant. You must adapt and refine your routines to keep your body challenged and prevent plateauing. This chapter will guide you in fine-tuning your resistance band exercises to ensure continuous progress.

When it comes to exercise, your body is an intelligent machine. It quickly adapts to routines. So, what felt hard last week may feel easy now. This is a sign to switch things up. We'll talk about how to adjust the intensity of your workouts.

One way to add intensity is by changing the band you use. Lighter bands are great to start with. You may need to use medium or heavy resistance bands as you get stronger.

Another way to fine-tune your routine is by adjusting the number of reps you do. If you've been doing 15 reps of an exercise and it's getting easier, try doing 20 reps. More reps mean more work for your muscles.

But take your time making all these changes at a time. It's best to change one thing at a time. This will let you see what works best for you.

Remember, our goal is to keep improving. But it's also to stay safe. Don't push so hard that you hurt yourself.

The key is to listen to your body. If something hurts, stop. If you're too tired to keep good form, stop. It's better to do fewer reps with good form than more reps with bad form.

Also, keep in mind that rest is part of the process. Your muscles need time to recover after a workout. Make sure to take a day off between workouts.

You can do light activities like walking or stretching on your rest days. This will keep your body moving without putting more stress on your muscles.

Now, let's talk about how to fit your workouts into your daily life. It's best to find a time that works for you and stick to it. This will make your workouts a habit.

Some people like to exercise in the morning. It wakes them up and gets it out of the way. Others prefer to exercise in the evening to wind down from the day.

ADVANCED RESISTANCE BAND WORKOUTS

"Your body is your most priceless possession. Take care of it." - Jack Lalane.

TRICEP KICKBACK

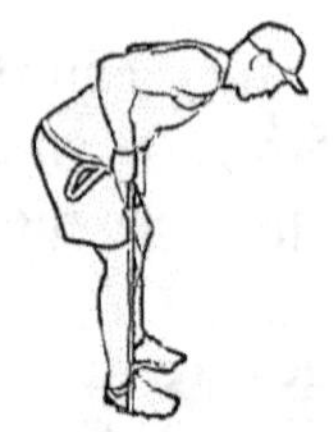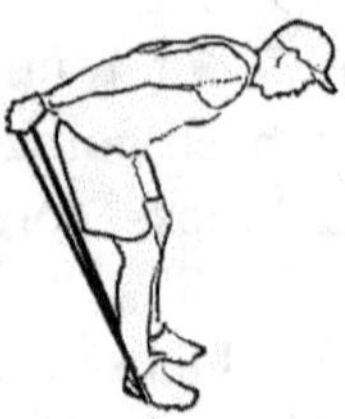

This exercise strengthens your triceps, enhancing upper body strength.

1. Stand on the band, feet shoulder-width apart.

2. Hold the other end of the band in one hand.

3. Bend forward slightly, keeping your back flat.

4. Extend your arm back, keeping your elbow stationary.

5. Repeat for ten reps on each side.

BANDED LEG LIFT

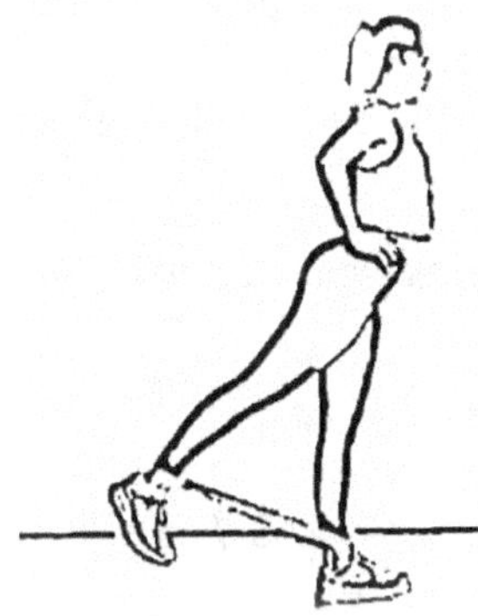

This exercise engages your glutes and hamstrings, supporting lower body strength and stability.

1. Tie the band around your ankles.

2. Stand tall, holding onto a chair for support if needed.

3. Lift one leg back, keeping your knee straight.

4. Return to the starting position.

5. Repeat for ten reps on each side.

These advanced resistance band workouts can help you maintain your strength, balance, and flexibility, all from the comfort of your home. By taking the time to practice these exercises, you are taking a vital step towards preserving your well-being and independence.

EXERCISES FOR DYNAMIC AND PLYOMETRIC MOVEMENTS FOR POWER AND STRENGTH

"It is exercise alone that supports the spirits, and keeps the mind in vigor." - Marcus Tullius Cicero.

Let's dive into five exercises that will help bring about the vigor that Cicero spoke of. These dynamic exercises involve plyometric movements, focusing on power and strength. They all use resistance bands, ensuring the challenge remains gentle yet effective for seniors.

BENT-OVER ROW

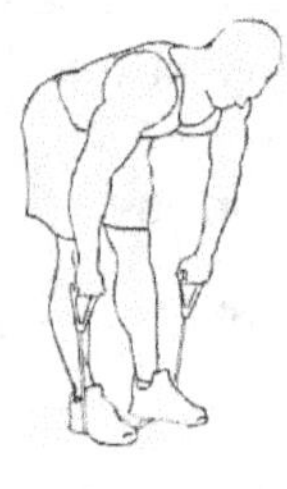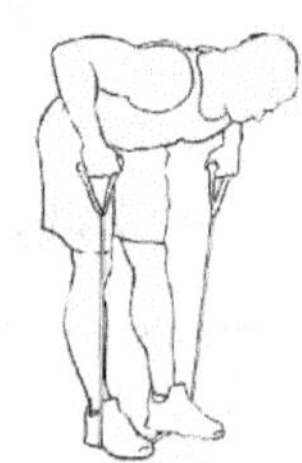

This exercise targets the muscles in your back, helping to improve posture and upper body strength.

1. Stand on the band with feet hip-width apart.

2. Bend at your waist, keeping your back flat.

3.   Hold the ends of the band, palms facing each other.

4.   Pull the band up towards your hips, keeping your elbows close to your body.

5.   Lower your arms slowly, maintaining resistance in the band.

6.   Repeat this exercise for 10-15 reps.

These exercises offer a dynamic and powerful way for seniors to maintain strength and vitality. They are simple and effective. Remember, the key to success is consistency. So, start slow, listen to your body, and gradually increase your intensity as you become stronger. Your body and mind will thank you for it.

COMBINING RESISTANCE BANDS WITH OTHER FITNESS TOOLS

Incorporating resistance bands with other fitness tools can expand your workout routine. It adds a fresh layer of challenge and variety. Bands are versatile, yet they also pair well with other fitness gear.

Dumbbells and resistance bands, for instance, work great together. Consider a bench press. You can add a resistance band to the barbell. This ups the pressure as you push upwards. For beginners, a light band is best. Intermediates can use a medium band. And the experienced, a heavy band.

The same logic applies to exercises like squats or deadlifts. For squats, loop a band around your thighs. This intensifies the lower body workout. Deadlifts, on the other hand, can be tweaked. Stand on the band and hold its ends along with the barbell. This adds resistance to the lift.

Moreover, resistance bands can also be combined with fitness balls. This enhances balance and core stability. For instance, try a ball squat. Stand on a band and hold its ends. Squat down onto a fitness ball. The band adds resistance as you rise.

Remember, these tools should enhance your workout, not complicate it. You must understand the mechanics of each exercise. The correct form is critical to prevent injury.

Yoga and Pilates enthusiasts can also benefit from resistance bands. They add intensity to poses and stretches. For a side stretch, hold a band overhead with both hands. Bend to one side, stretching the band over your head. This deepens the side stretch.

Similarly, a band can add resistance to leg and arm movements in Pilates. It intensifies the workout and aids in better muscle toning.

Resistance bands are also helpful in cardio workouts. They add an element of strength training to your aerobic exercise. For example, during step-ups, use a band. Tie it around your ankles. This adds resistance as you step up and down. It works your leg muscles more.

PERIODIZATION AND LONG-TERM PROGRESSION

"The key to long-term success is the regular practice of a lifestyle that includes physical activity." - Kenneth H. Cooper.

Periodization is crucial in fitness. It breaks down the training plan into periods. Each period has a goal. It is an intelligent way to train. It can prevent overtraining. It keeps the workouts from getting stale.

The first part of periodization is the macrocycle. It is the longest of the three cycles, lasting several months or even a year. It is the big picture of the training program.

Next is the mesocycle. It lasts for several weeks to a few months. It is a specific block of training designed to achieve a particular goal.

Finally, the microcycle is typically a week. It details specific workouts for the week.

Long-term progression is also crucial. It is the steady increase in workout intensity. It helps to avoid plateaus. It also helps to prevent injuries.

Chapter 8:

LIFESTYLE AND WELL-BEING

"Health is a state of the body. Wellness is a state of being." - J. Stanford.

Our well-being is a state of health, happiness, and prosperity. It encompasses our physical health, mental health, and our sense of life satisfaction. It's not just about being free from illness but about leading a balanced and fulfilling life.

Research shows that our lifestyle choices can significantly influence our well-being. It can affect our physical health, mental health, and lifespan. Certain lifestyle behaviors, such as regular physical activity, a balanced diet, adequate sleep, and avoiding harmful habits like smoking or excessive drinking, are crucial for maintaining our health and well-being.

Resistance band exercises can play a significant role in enhancing our lifestyle and well-being. Regular resistance band exercises can improve physical health by strengthening muscles, improving flexibility, enhancing balance, and boosting cardio fitness. It may also aid in weight management and prevent various health conditions such as heart disease, diabetes, and osteoporosis.

Resistance band exercises are not just beneficial for our physical health. Regular exercise can also enhance our mental well-being. It can improve mood, reduce stress, anxiety, and depression, and boost self-esteem. It can enhance cognitive function, improve sleep quality, and contribute to a greater sense of well-being.

INCORPORATING RESISTANCE BAND EXERCISES INTO DAILY ROUTINES

This quote rings true when we think about fitness. And in this case, we're talking about resistance band exercises.

Resistance bands are not just another fitness fad. They are a powerful tool for staying active, especially for seniors. Many fitness experts and studies, such as one from the Journal of Physical Therapy Science, have noted the positive impacts of resistance band exercises.

First off, resistance bands are portable. You can pack them in your bag and take them wherever you go. This means you can exercise anytime, anywhere. They're perfect for home workouts, park exercises, or even during travel.

Second, these bands are versatile. You can use them for a wide range of exercises. Resistance bands can work out different muscle groups, from arm curls to leg lifts. This makes them a great addition to your daily routine.

PROPER NUTRITION AND HYDRATION FOR OPTIMAL FITNESS

One of the core elements of a successful fitness plan, especially for seniors, is proper nutrition. What we eat and drink is vital in how we feel, move, and age. It's about more than just the exercises we do with resistance bands or other equipment.

Our bodies need fuel, and the quality of that fuel matters. It's like a car. If you put in low-quality gas, the car won't run as smoothly and might even end up with engine problems. The same goes for our bodies. Our bodies only perform well if we feed them healthy, low-quality foods.

So, what does proper nutrition look like? It's a balanced diet of fruits, vegetables, lean proteins, whole grains, and healthy fats. These foods provide the nutrients our bodies need to function at their best. They give us energy, help us recover after workouts, and strengthen our bodies.

Fruits and vegetables are packed with vitamins and minerals. They also have fiber, which can help keep our digestive system healthy. Lean proteins, like fish, chicken, and legumes, help build and repair muscles. Whole grains, such as brown rice and oatmeal, give us energy. Healthy fats, like those found in avocados and olive oil, support our heart health.

Hydration is also crucial for optimal fitness. Our bodies need water to function. It helps regulate our body temperature, lubricate our joints, and transport nutrients to our cells. When we exercise, we lose water through sweat. So, drinking plenty of water before, during, and after workouts is essential to stay hydrated.

Now, let's talk about portion control. It's not just about what we eat but how much we eat. Even healthy foods can lead to weight gain if we consume them in large amounts. So, it's essential to pay attention to portion sizes. A simple rule of thumb is to fill half your plate with fruits and vegetables, a quarter with lean proteins, and a quarter with whole grains.

Eating healthy doesn't mean you have to give up your favorite foods. It's about making smart choices most of the time. If you love chocolate, for example, you don't have to cut it out completely. But instead of eating a whole bar, have a small piece as a treat.

Remember, everyone's nutritional needs are different. What works for one person might not work for another. So, it's essential to listen to your body and adjust your diet as needed. If you need help with what or how much to eat, consider consulting a nutritionist or dietitian. They can provide personalized advice based on your health and fitness goals.

In conclusion, proper nutrition and hydration are essential to optimal fitness. Eating a balanced diet, staying hydrated, and paying attention to portion sizes can fuel your body with what it needs to stay healthy and strong. Combined with regular exercise, like resistance band workouts, proper nutrition can help you improve your balance, strength, flexibility, and overall well-being.

MANAGING STRESS AND IMPROVING MENTAL WELL-BEING

"It's not stress that kills us; it is our reaction to it." - Hans Selye.

Stress is a part of life. It can be a motivator, pushing us to reach our goals. But too much stress can hurt us. It can make us feel overwhelmed and hurt our mental health. Managing stress is critical to improving mental well-being. This is especially true for seniors, who may face unique stressors such as health issues, loss of loved ones, or changes in living situations.

One of the ways to manage stress is through regular exercise. Exercise releases chemicals in your brain that make you feel happier and more relaxed. It can also help you sleep better, which can have a positive effect on your mood and stress levels.

MAINTAINING AN ACTIVE LIFESTYLE

"Age is no barrier. It's a limitation you put on your mind." - Jackie Joyner-Kersee.

Staying active as we age is vital to our well-being. It helps improve our physical health and keeps our minds sharp. But how can we maintain an active lifestyle in our later years? The answer is through regular exercise. One of the most influential and accessible forms of exercise is resistance band training.

Resistance bands are an excellent tool for seniors. They are easy to use, affordable, and can be used anywhere, at any time. They offer low-impact exercise, making them perfect for seniors with joint issues or mobility challenges.

OVERCOMING COMMON OBSTACLES AND CHALLENGES

"Strength doesn't come from what you can do, it comes from overcoming the things you once thought you couldn't." - Rikki Rogers.

Obstacles and challenges are part of life. Even more so in our senior years. They can make us feel stuck. But we can overcome them. We can move beyond them. One way to do this is through exercising with resistance bands. These simple tools offer a way to regain strength, balance, and flexibility, enhancing our overall well-being.

Take limited body mobility, for example. It can make daily activities a struggle. But exercises with resistance bands can help. They can allow us to regain our independence. They can make us feel more capable and confident.

Resistance bands are also a time-efficient exercise option. You don't need to spend hours at a gym. You don't need to invest in heavy, space-consuming equipment. All you need is a band. And a little bit of time each day.

Balance and stability are other common issues. They can lead to falls and injuries. They can make us fear physical activities. But resistance bands can help here, too. They can improve our balance. They can make us feel more stable and secure on our feet.

This book is not just about exercises. It's about improving our quality of life. It's about being able to do the things we love. It's about feeling strong, flexible, and balanced. It's about living a healthy life.

There are many other exercises we can do with resistance bands. Each of them targets different muscle groups. Each of them helps us in different ways. They can all help us overcome common obstacles and challenges.

We're always young enough to exercise. We're always young enough to improve our health. We're always young enough to overcome challenges. And with resistance bands, we can do it from the comfort of our homes. We can do it at our own pace. We can do it in a way that suits us.

SEEKING SUPPORT AND ACCOUNTABILITY

"When 'I' is replaced by 'We', even 'illness' becomes 'wellness'." - Malcolm X

Starting a new fitness routine takes work, especially as a senior. But you're not alone. One of the best ways to stay motivated is to seek support and accountability. It's a vital part of the process.

Support can come from many sources. It might be a spouse, a child, a friend, or a fitness trainer. They could be your gym buddy or someone checking in with you regularly. They'll be there to cheer you on and to help you stay on track.

Accountability is also essential. It means having someone who holds you to your commitment. They'll ask about your progress and encourage you to keep going. It's not about judgment but about helping you stay focused on your goals.

Being accountable to someone gives you a sense of responsibility. It pushes you to do your best. You don't want to let them down. It's a powerful motivator.

An accountability partner can also provide feedback. They can help you adjust your routine if it's too hard or too easy. They can spot when you're struggling and give you the boost you need to keep going.

It's also important to remember that you're not just seeking support and accountability for yourself. You're also providing it for the other person. It's a two-way street. You're in this together.

Remember, it's okay to ask for help. We all need a little push sometimes. It's not a sign of weakness but a step towards strength.

The beauty of seeking support and accountability is that it helps you stick to your fitness routine and strengthens your relationships. It's a way to connect with others on a deeper level. It's a way to share your journey and to grow together.

Now, you might be wondering how to find an accountability partner. It could be anyone who shares your fitness goals. It could be someone who's also a senior or someone younger. It could be someone you meet at a local community center or online.

Once you've found your partner, set clear expectations. Discuss your goals and how you will help each other achieve them. Decide how often you're going to check in with each other. And most importantly, make sure it's someone you trust and feel comfortable with.

Resistance band exercises aren't just about physical strength. They're also about mental strength. They're about resilience and determination. And having someone by your side can make all the difference.

So, don't hesitate. Reach out to someone today. Start your journey towards better health together. Remember, it's not just about the destination but also the journey. And it's a journey best shared with others.

The support and accountability you seek today will lead to the success you achieve tomorrow. They're the pillars holding you up as you work towards your fitness goals. They're the steppingstones towards a healthier, happier you.

Remember, every step counts, no matter how small. Every rep matters, no matter how light the resistance band may be. It's not about how fast you go but about the fact that you're moving forward.

With the proper support and accountability, you'll not only reach your fitness goals, but you'll also enjoy the journey towards them. You'll turn challenges into victories, doubts into confidence, and goals into realities.

So, as you begin your fitness journey with resistance bands, remember to seek support and accountability. They're your allies in your quest for better health, balance, and well-being. And with them by your side, you're sure to succeed.

After all, fitness is not a solo act. It's a team effort. It's about pushing each other to be better, stronger, and healthier. It's about celebrating each other's successes and picking each other up when we fall.

So, take the first step today. Seek support. Seek accountability. And together, transform your "illness" into "wellness." As Malcolm X wisely said, it's all about replacing the 'I' with 'We'. So, let's do this together. Let's embrace the power of 'We.'

CELEBRATING YOUR ACHIEVEMENTS AND SETBACKS

"Success is not the key to happiness. Happiness is the key to success. If you love what you are doing, you will be successful." - Albert Schweitzer.

Life is a beautiful mix of ups and downs. As we age, we may find our bodies less nimble or our strength less robust. Yet, in these moments of struggle, we can find our courage and tenacity. It is from these challenges that we can recognize and celebrate our achievements.

Let's start with our achievements. Each time you complete an exercise, it's an achievement. Every time you use your resistance band, you're scoring a win. It might not seem like a big deal, but it is. You're taking steps to improve your health. You're working on your mobility, balance, and strength. These are all victories worthy of celebration.

Remember, it's not about being the best. It's about being better than you were yesterday. It's about showing up, even when you don't like it. It's about picking up your resistance band and doing your exercises. Each small step you take is a giant leap for your health.

But what about setbacks? Yes, they will happen. There will be days when you don't feel up to exercising. There might be times when you can't do an exercise you were able to do before. These are not failures. They're just part of the process.

Setbacks allow us to learn and grow. They show us where we need to improve. They teach us to be patient with ourselves. And most importantly, they remind us that we are human.

It's important not to dwell on these setbacks. Instead, see them as steppingstones to your success. They don't define you, but they can help shape you. They provide invaluable insights and experiences you can use to better yourself.

One of the most beautiful aspects of life is its unpredictability. The same goes for our fitness journey. Some days will be easy, and some will be tough. But each day offers us a chance to grow, learn, and become stronger.

Use your achievements as motivation to keep going. Use your setbacks as lessons to become better. Remember, you're becoming stronger, healthier, and more resilient with every step you take, exercise, and resistance band you use. And that is something to celebrate.

Our bodies may change as we age, but our spirit doesn't have to. We can still stay active, healthy, and, most importantly, happy. We can make the most of these golden years by caring for our health and celebrating each achievement, no matter how small.

Chapter 9:

NUTRITION AND RECOVERY STRATEGIES

Nutrition plays a significant role in our health. It fuels our bodies for workouts. It also helps us recover after. For seniors, getting the proper nutrients is essential. It helps maintain strength and flexibility. It also aids in recovery after exercise.

Protein is a crucial nutrient for seniors. It helps with muscle recovery. After a workout, protein helps repair the muscles. This aids in faster recovery. Seniors should aim for a diet rich in lean protein. Eggs, chicken, and fish are good sources.

Carbohydrates are also essential. They provide energy for workouts. Complex carbohydrates are the best. They release energy slowly. This keeps energy levels stable. Examples of complex carbs include whole grains, brown rice, and oats.

Fruits and vegetables are essential, too. They are rich in vitamins and minerals. These nutrients aid in recovery. They also boost the immune system. Seniors should aim for a diverse range of fruits and vegetables. This ensures they get a variety of nutrients.

Hydration is vital for seniors. Water helps in nutrient absorption. It also aids in digestion. Seniors should drink enough water throughout the day. They should also replace fluids lost during workouts.

Recovery strategies are also essential. These help the body heal after workouts. One effective strategy is rest. After a workout, seniors should take time to rest. This allows the body to recover.

Stretching is another strategy. It helps relax the muscles. This reduces muscle tension after workouts. Seniors should include light stretching in their routine. This aids in recovery.

Sleep is a crucial recovery strategy. It allows the body to repair itself. Seniors should aim for quality sleep. This ensures they wake up refreshed and ready for the next workout.

A balanced diet, proper hydration, and effective recovery strategies are essential. They aid in post-workout recovery for seniors. They also improve overall health. This helps seniors maintain their strength and flexibility. It also enhances their well-being.

GRILLED CHICKEN BREAST

"The only real stumbling block is fear of failure. In cooking, you've got to have a what-the-hell attitude." - Julia Child.

Grilled chicken breast is a versatile and healthy protein source. It's a go-to for many home cooks. When examined right, it is juicy, tender, and flavorful. Though simple, there's an art to grilling chicken breast. Let's walk through it.

Start by choosing a good chicken breast. A fresh, organic, and boneless cut is best. It should be firm to the touch and pinkish. Avoid any with a solid or off smell. Next, prep your chicken. Clean it under cold running water. Pat dry with paper towels.

Now, let's talk about marinating. It works magic on chicken breasts, making them flavorful and moist. Use olive oil, lemon juice, garlic, herbs, and spices. Let the chicken sit in this mix for at least 30 minutes. But if you can, leave it overnight. More time equals more flavor.

Once marinated, it's time to grill. Preheat your grill to medium-high heat. You want it hot enough to sear the chicken and keep it juicy. When the grill is ready, place your chicken breasts on it. Cook each side for about six to seven minutes.

How do you tell when your chicken is done? A cooking thermometer is your best bet. Insert it into the thickest part of the breast. It should read 165 degrees Fahrenheit. You can slice into the chicken if you don't have a thermometer. The juice should be clear, not pink.

Grilled chicken breast is not just tasty; it's packed with nutrients. It's low in fat and high in protein. It's also a great source of vitamins B6, B12, D, calcium, iron, and zinc. It's good for your heart health and helps build muscle.

In terms of serving, grilled chicken breast is super flexible. Slice it up for salads, tacos, or pasta. Serve it whole with a side of veggies. Use it in sandwiches or wraps. The options are endless.

Finally, remember that grilling is an art. It takes time and practice to get it right. Don't be disheartened if your first few tries don't turn out perfectly. Keep at it. With time, you'll master the art of grilling chicken breasts.

QUINOA OR BROWN RICE

"Let food be thy medicine and medicine be thy food." - Hippocrates

When we speak of food as an energy source and a tool for well-being, grains come to mind. Grains are a vital part of our diet, offering a variety of benefits. Two grains that stand out are quinoa and brown rice. Each has unique qualities and advantages that can help seniors maintain a healthy lifestyle and exercise routines.

Quinoa, often referred to as a superfood, is a complete protein. It contains all nine essential amino acids that we need from our diet. It's also high in fiber and rich in vitamins and minerals. These nutrients play a crucial part in muscle recovery and overall health.

Brown rice is a whole grain, full of fiber. Fiber helps to keep the digestive system healthy and can aid in weight management. It's also a good source of vitamins and minerals, particularly B vitamins. These vitamins are essential in energy production and vital to maintaining an active lifestyle.

It's important to note that each grain has a unique taste and texture. Quinoa has a nutty flavor and a slightly crunchy texture, while brown rice is slightly chewy with a mild, nutty flavor. These different tastes can add variety to your meals and keep your diet interesting.

When preparing quinoa or brown rice, remember a few things. Both grains require rinsing before cooking to remove any dust or residues. They should also be cooked in a pot with a lid to ensure even cooking.

Quinoa cooks faster than brown rice. It usually takes 15 minutes for quinoa to cook, compared to 45 minutes for brown rice. This difference in cooking time can be helpful when planning meals. Quick meals can benefit from quinoa's fast cooking time, while meals requiring more preparation can incorporate brown rice.

One of the benefits of these grains is their versatility. They can be used in a variety of dishes. Quinoa can be used in salads, soups, stews, and breakfast cereal. Brown rice can be used in stir-fries, soups, salads, and as a side dish.

STEAMED VEGETABLES

Vegetables are packed with essential nutrients that our bodies need to function at their best. They are rich in vitamins, minerals, and fiber, which can help reduce the risk of many health conditions, including heart disease, stroke, and certain types of cancer.

Steaming is a cooking method that can help retain the maximum nutrients in vegetables. Unlike other cooking methods, such as boiling or frying, steaming does not require the vegetables to be submerged in water or oil. This means that the nutrients in the vegetables are not lost through leaching or absorption.

Steaming vegetables is a quick and easy process. You only need a steamer basket and a pot with a tight-fitting lid. Simply fill the pot with a small amount of water, place the vegetables in the steamer basket, and then place the basket in the pot. Cover the pot and bring the water to a boil. The steam from the boiling water will cook the vegetables, preserving their nutrients and vibrant colors.

In addition to being nutrient-dense, steamed vegetables are also low in calories. This makes them an excellent choice for seniors trying to maintain a healthy weight. They are also easy to chew and digest, which can benefit seniors with teeth or digestive system difficulties.

Many different types of vegetables can be steamed. Some popular choices include broccoli, carrots, zucchini, and green beans. However, any vegetable can be steamed. Experiment with different types and combinations of vegetables to find your favorites.

Not only are steamed vegetables nutritious and easy to prepare, but they are also versatile. They can be served as a side dish, added to salads, or used as ingredients in various recipes. For example, steamed vegetables can make a stir-fry, a soup, or a casserole.

GREEK YOGURT WITH BERRIES

Greek yogurt and berries, a powerhouse combo, serve as an excellent meal for seniors. It's not just about the taste. This combo is a nutritional goldmine. It's packed with protein, probiotics, antioxidants, and fiber. It's easy for seniors to prepare and consume.

Greek yogurt is a protein-rich food. It's an excellent source for seniors who need to maintain muscle mass. It's thicker and creamier than regular yogurt. It offers more protein and fewer carbs. This helps to keep seniors full and satisfied.

Berries, on the other hand, are full of antioxidants. They help protect the body from damage by harmful molecules called free radicals. Berries like blueberries, strawberries, raspberries, and blackberries are rich in vitamins A, C, and E. They also have a high fiber content.

Combining Greek yogurt with berries makes for a tasty, nutritious meal. It's a good option for breakfast or a snack. It can even be a dessert substitute for seniors with a sweet tooth. It requires minimal prep time. Just a cup of Greek yogurt and a handful of berries are enough.

This meal combo is also versatile. Seniors can mix and match different types of berries. They can also add nuts or granola for extra crunch and fiber. Honey or maple syrup can be drizzled on top for added sweetness.

The probiotics in Greek yogurt are beneficial for gut health. They help balance the gut microbiota. This is crucial for digestion and overall health. A healthy gut has been linked to a robust immune system. For seniors, this is essential for disease prevention.

The fiber from the berry's aids in digestion, too. It helps prevent constipation, a common issue among seniors. Regular bowel movements contribute to a feeling of well-being.

This meal also contributes to bone health. Greek yogurt is a good source of calcium. This mineral is essential for bone strength. It helps prevent osteoporosis, a condition common in seniors.

Berries, particularly strawberries, are high in vitamin K. This vitamin also plays a role in bone health. It helps the body use calcium to build bones.

Greek yogurt with berries is a heart-healthy meal. The antioxidants in berries help lower blood pressure. They also reduce the risk of heart disease. Greek yogurt has been found to have similar effects.

This meal also helps maintain healthy skin. The antioxidants in berries protect the skin from damage. They help keep the skin looking youthful. The protein in Greek yogurt aids in tissue repair. This includes the skin tissue.

POST-WORKOUT NUTRITION

"Food is the fuel that helps athletes perform their best." - Unknown

After a workout, your body is in a state of repair. It needs the proper nutrients to recover. The food you eat post-exercise plays a critical role in this process. It can distinguish between a productive workout and one that leaves you feeling drained.

Protein is key. It helps with muscle recovery. It also aids in the growth of new tissue. You need to include enough protein in your diet. There are many sources of protein. These include lean meat, fish, and eggs. Plant-based sources include beans, lentils, and tofu.

Carbohydrates are also essential. They replenish the energy lost during the workout. Fruits, whole grains, and vegetables are good sources of carbs. These foods provide the body with fiber. Fiber aids in digestion and keeps you feeling full longer.

Hydration is another critical factor. It is easy to get dehydrated during a workout. Drinking enough water helps replace the fluids lost. It also aids in digestion and absorption of nutrients.

Post-workout meals should be balanced. They should contain a mix of protein, carbs, and healthy fats. Eating a meal within 45 minutes of your workout is ideal. This is the time when your body is most receptive to nutrients.

Snacks can also be beneficial. They provide a quick source of energy. Nuts, yogurt, and fruit are good options. These foods are easy to digest. They provide the body with the nutrients it needs.

Supplements can also aid in recovery. Protein shakes and bars are popular choices. They can provide a quick and convenient source of protein. However, they should not replace whole foods. Whole foods offer a variety of nutrients. These nutrients work together to support overall health.

Remember that everyone is different. What works for one person may only work for one person. Experiment with other foods and timing. Find what works best for you.

Remember to listen to your body. It will tell you what it needs. If you feel tired or weak, you may need more nutrients. If you feel full and satisfied, you may be eating enough.

Post-workout nutrition is not just about what you eat. It's also about when you eat. Timing is crucial. Eating at the right time can optimize recovery. It can also improve performance in future workouts.

HYDRATION TIPS

"Water is life's matter and matrix, mother and medium. There is no life without water." - Albert Szent-Gyorgyi.

Hydration is a vital part of our health. Yet, our thirst may dull as we age, leading to inadequate water intake. This section of the book will guide you through the importance of hydration during your home workouts and provide valuable tips to ensure you stay well-hydrated.

As we age, our bodies' water content decreases. Therefore, it becomes even more crucial to maintain hydration, especially during physical activities. Water is the primary component of all cells in the body. It helps regulate body temperature, lubricates joints, aids digestion, and is essential for nutrient absorption. We may experience fatigue, dizziness, or even more severe dehydration symptoms without adequate hydration.

While exercising, your body loses water through sweat. Even gentle exercises such as resistance band workouts can lead to fluid loss. Therefore, drinking water before, during, and after training is essential. But how much water should you consume? The answer depends on the intensity and duration of your workout.

A good rule of thumb is to drink at least two cups of water two hours before your workout. Aim for half a cup to one cup during the exercise every 15 to 20 minutes. After your workout, drink at least two to three cups of water. Remember, these are general guidelines, and individual needs may vary based on several factors, including age, gender, weight, and overall health.

Aside from water, consider drinks with electrolytes, such as sports or coconut water. Electrolytes, including sodium, potassium, and magnesium, are crucial for muscle function and maintaining fluid balance in your body. During exercise, they are lost through sweat, and replenishing them can aid recovery.

You might wonder, "What about other beverages like tea, coffee, or soda?" While these drinks contain water, there are better options for hydration during workouts. Caffeinated beverages like coffee and tea can act as diuretics, promoting fluid loss. On the other hand, soda is high in sugar and can lead to weight gain if consumed regularly.

SLEEP AND MUSCLE RECOVERY

"Sleep is that golden chain that ties health and our bodies together." - Thomas Dekker

---

When we consider muscle recovery, sleep plays a crucial role. While we rest, our bodies work hard to rebuild and repair our muscles.

In the fitness world, we often pay attention to workouts and diet. But we should remember that sleep is equally essential for muscle recovery. It's during sleep that our bodies repair muscle tissue damaged during workouts. This process is critical for muscle growth and strength.

Resistance band exercises, as discussed in this book, are quite beneficial. But, without proper sleep, our muscles can't fully recover. It's like building a house without allowing the cement to dry. Rest is when our muscles grow and heal, preparing us for the next day's activities.

Deep sleep, in particular, plays a significant role in muscle recovery. Our bodies release human growth hormone (HGH) during this sleep phase. This hormone is crucial for muscle growth and repair. If we don't sleep enough, our bodies can't release enough HGH, hindering muscle recovery.

Studies have shown that lack of sleep can slow down muscle recovery. So, if you're not sleeping well, your muscles may not recover fully from your resistance band exercises. This lack of recovery can lead to muscle fatigue and even injuries. So, make sure you're getting enough sleep every night.

Sleep also helps our bodies manage inflammation. When we work out, our muscles experience some inflammation. This inflammation is a normal part of the muscle recovery process. However, it can slow down muscle recovery if our bodies don't manage it well. Sleep helps our bodies fight this inflammation, promoting quicker muscle recovery.

Furthermore, sleep helps our bodies manage stress. When we're stressed, our bodies produce a hormone called cortisol. This hormone can slow down muscle recovery. But when we sleep, our bodies can manage stress better, reducing cortisol production.

Nutrition is another critical factor in muscle recovery. Protein, in particular, is crucial for muscle repair. When we sleep, our bodies can better absorb the protein consumed during the day. This process helps our muscles recover and grow stronger.

In conclusion, sleep is an essential component of muscle recovery. Get enough sleep if you're doing resistance band exercises or any other workout. This rest will help your muscles recover and prepare for the next day's activities.

Sleep is not a luxury. It's a necessity for our bodies, especially for muscle recovery. So, make sure you're getting enough of it. And remember, it's not just about the quantity of sleep but also the quality. Strive to get deep, restful sleep every night.

Remember, sleep is a critical part of your exercise routine. It's during sleep that our muscles recover and grow stronger. So, pay attention to it. Make sleep a priority in your fitness journey; you'll see better results from your resistance band exercises.

To ensure good sleep, maintain a healthy sleep routine. Try to go to bed and wake up simultaneously every day. Avoid screens before bedtime, as they can interfere with your sleep. And make sure your bedroom is dark, quiet, and relaxed.

LISTEN TO YOUR BODY

"The body is a temple; we must look after it."

This ancient adage might seem cliché, but its wisdom has stood the test of time for a reason. As we age, maintaining our physical health becomes even more critical. A significant part of caring for our bodies involves tuning into what they're telling us.

Our bodies communicate with us in a variety of ways. They tell us when we're hungry, tired, or in pain. They alert us to danger and respond to pleasure. Understanding these signals and responding to them appropriately is crucial, especially as we get older.

One of the most common indicators our bodies give us is fatigue. If you're feeling tired, it's essential to rest. Pushing through fatigue can lead to injury or other health issues. Similarly, if you're experiencing pain during exercise, it's crucial to stop and address the issue. Pain is the body's way of alerting us that something is wrong.

As we age, our bodies also tend to take longer to recover from physical activity. Be encouraged if you can't bounce back as quickly as you used to. It's a normal part of aging and doesn't mean you're not progressing. Slower recovery times can be a sign that your body is working hard to adapt to the new demands you're placing on it.

Another important aspect of listening to your body involves understanding your limits. Getting caught up in the progress and pushing yourself too hard is easy. If you're feeling lightheaded, dizzy, or unusually short of breath during a workout, it's time to take a break. Pushing your body past its limits can lead to injury and set you back in your fitness journey.

In addition to physical signals, our bodies also communicate with us emotionally. Exercise is known to boost mood and reduce feelings of anxiety and depression. If you're feeling down, a gentle workout is what you need to lift your spirits. Similarly, physical activity can help calm your mind if you're anxious or stressed.

Finally, it's important to remember that listening to your body is a skill that takes time to develop. It involves paying close attention to and responding to your body's signals respectfully. It's about balancing pushing yourself to grow and not causing harm.

Chapter 10:

TROUBLESHOOTING AND AVOIDING PLATEAUS

"The only way to do great work is to love what you do." - Steve Jobs

Resistance band exercises can be a game changer in improving our balance, strength, flexibility, and overall well-being. However, there may be times when you hit a plateau. Don't worry; we'll get through it together.

Plateaus happen when your body gets used to the same workout routine. Your muscles have a memory. They get used to the exercises you do. When you hit a plateau, it's a sign that you need to change things up.

If you're not seeing the progress you want, it might be time to switch your routine. Try some new exercises. Change the order of your practice. Or increase the resistance of the bands.

Another reason for hitting a plateau could be a lack of rest. Our bodies need time to recover. That's when real growth happens. Make sure you're giving your body the rest it needs.

Nutrition also plays a crucial role in our fitness goals. It will only perform at its best if you're fueling your body right. Make sure to eat a balanced diet. Drink plenty of water. And avoid processed foods.

Consider working with a fitness expert. They can help you break through your plateau. They can guide you on the correct exercises. And they can make sure you're doing them correctly.

Remember, consistency is critical. Keep showing up. Keep doing the work. And the results will follow.

On the other hand, we don't only plateau because we're doing the same workouts. Sometimes, we plateau because we're not pushing ourselves hard enough.

Don't be afraid to challenge yourself. Increase the resistance of your bands. Or try some advanced exercises. Just make sure to do it gradually. And always listen to your body.

Another factor that can lead to plateaus is stress. Stress can hurt our fitness goals. It can lead to muscle tension. And it can hinder our recovery. Try to manage your stress levels. Meditation and deep breathing exercises can help.

PLATEAU BUSTING STRATEGIES

"The secret of getting ahead is getting started." - Mark Twain

Getting fit is a process. It takes time, effort, and patience. You've been doing great on your fitness journey, but we may hit a fitness plateau as we age. This is where progress seems to stop, no matter how hard we try. But don't worry; we can break through this plateau with some practical strategies.

The first strategy is to change your routine. Your body adapts to exercises over time, and it becomes more efficient. When this happens, the same exercises burn fewer calories and build less muscle. To counter this, mix up your workouts. Use your resistance band in new ways. This shocks your body into adapting again, which boosts progress.

The second strategy is to increase intensity. If your workouts feel easy, they need to be more challenging. To improve, you have to push your limits. Add more resistance to your band or quicken your pace. Remember, always listen to your body, and don't overdo it.

The third strategy is to focus on nutrition. Exercise is crucial, but so is what you eat. Your body needs the right fuel to perform and recover. Ensure you eat a balanced diet with plenty of protein, fruits, and vegetables. Stay hydrated, too. Water is essential for all bodily functions, including muscle recovery.

Next, consider adding some variety to your routine. This doesn't only mean changing the exercises you do but also the type of exercise. If you've focused solely on strength training, add some cardio. Walking is a great start. It's low-impact and can be done anywhere. Cardio is excellent for heart health and aids in weight management.

Another effective strategy is rest. Yes, rest! Your body needs time to recover and build muscle. If you're constantly pushing yourself without giving your body time to heal, you may see a decrease in performance.

Finally, remember to stay consistent. Fitness is a journey, not a destination. There will be ups and downs, progress, and plateaus. But don't give up. Keep going, keep striving. Consistency is vital in any endeavor, including fitness.

ACHIEVING YOUR FITNESS GOALS

"The only way to achieve the impossible is to believe it is possible." - Charles Kingsleigh.

In the pursuit of physical wellness, we often encounter barriers. Age, lack of mobility, or fear of injury can hold us back. Yet, it's crucial to remember that fitness is attainable regardless of age or physical limitations.

This section will guide you through the process of achieving your fitness goals. You may wonder, "Can I, at my age, really improve my strength, balance, and flexibility?" The answer is a resounding "Yes!" The key lies in utilizing the right tools and techniques catered to your unique needs.

You must remember that fitness is not a race; it's a steady journey towards better health. Therefore, start slowly and gradually increase your exercise's intensity and frequency. Listen to your body and adjust your workouts accordingly. This approach ensures that you stay safe while still challenging yourself physically.

Additionally, consistency is critical in achieving your fitness goals. Regular workout routines are more effective than sporadic and intensive exercise sessions. Aim to incorporate resistance band exercises into your daily routine, making them as common as eating or sleeping.

It's also essential to maintain a positive mindset. Aging and physical limitations can often lead to frustration. However, remember that progress is still progress, no matter how small. Celebrate each milestone, and don't get disheartened by slow progress or setbacks.

Moreover, don't hesitate to seek professional guidance. Working with a physical therapist or a personal trainer can provide personalized advice and exercise routines. They can ensure your workouts are safe, effective, and tailored to your needs.

Conclusion

In this book, we have walked through the world of resistance band exercises for seniors. We have seen how these simple, yet effective exercises can enhance balance, strength, flexibility, and overall well-being. The book offers a treasure trove of exercises, each carefully planned and described. Each exercise has been designed to be easy to follow and perform at home, using resistance bands suitable for different experience levels.

The importance of maintaining physical health as we age cannot be overstated. Limited mobility, poor balance, and the inability to engage in everyday activities can severely impact the quality of life. But, as we discovered throughout this book, these challenges can be mitigated. With resistance band exercises, seniors can improve their strength, enhance their flexibility, and restore their balance. This not only leads to increased independence but also infuses a renewed sense of confidence.

We explored a variety of exercises, each accompanied by a detailed description and step-by-step instructions. Each exercise was categorized according to the experience level - beginner, intermediate, or experienced - and allocated a suitable type of resistance band.

In conclusion, the journey to improved health and well-being must be manageable. It can start at home, with a resistance band and the will to change positively. The exercises presented in this book offer a safe, efficient, and enjoyable way for seniors to regain their vitality and independence.

Remember, each step towards better health is a more fulfilling life. The tools are now in your hands. It's time to put them to use. Start your resistance band workout today and witness the transformational power of consistent, mindful exercise.

If you find this book helpful, please leave a review on Amazon. Your feedback is invaluable and will help others in their journey towards improved health and well-being.

Embrace the power of resistance band exercises and let the journey to better health begin!

Index of Exercises

If you've just finished reading my book, I want to express my heartfelt gratitude for taking the time to explore its pages. Your insights, opinions, and feedback are incredibly valuable, not only to me but also to other potential readers who are considering diving into the world I've crafted.

Sharing your thoughts in an Amazon review can make a world of difference. Your words have the power to inspire and guide fellow readers, helping them discover the magic and insights that lie within the book's covers. Whether you were captivated by the characters, enlightened by the ideas, or moved by the story, your review can be a beacon, drawing more readers into this literary journey.

Your honest and thoughtful review can provide a window into your own experience, helping others decide if this book is the right fit for them. It's a simple yet profound way to pay it forward, contributing to the growth of a vibrant community of readers and storytellers.

So, please consider leaving a review on Amazon today. Your words can create ripples of impact, connecting you with fellow readers and writers, and together, we can continue to celebrate the beauty and power of literature. Thank you for being a part of this incredible journey, and for sharing your voice with the world.